Workbook to Accompany

Clinical Application of Blood Gases

Fifth Edition

by Paul Mathews and Barbara A. Ludwig

Workbook to Accompany

Clinical Application of Blood Gases

Fifth Edition

Paul Mathews, EdS, RRT, FCCM
Associate Professor

Barbara A. Ludwig, MA, RRT
Assistant Professor
Acting Chair

Department of Respiratory Care Education
School of Allied Health
The University of Kansas Medical Center
Kansas City, Kansas

Mosby

St. Louis Baltimore Berlin Boston Carlsbad Chicago London Madrid
Naples New York Philadelphia Sydney Tokyo Toronto

Mosby
Dedicated to Publishing Excellence

Editor: James F. Shanahan
Developmental Editor: Jennifer Roche
Manuscript Editor: Susan Warrington
Cover design: Brian Hill
Interior design: Ken Wendling

Printed in the United States of America
Composition by Wordbench

Mosby–Year Book, Inc.
11830 Westline Industrial Drive
St. Louis, MO 63146

ISBN 0-8151-7586-8
23839

1 2 3 4 5 6 7 8 9 0 98 97 96 95 94 93

Dedication

The authors wish to dedicate this workbook to Donald F. Egan, M.D., and Hugh S. Mathewson, M.D.: Mentors, Colleagues and Friends.

Learning is not a destination — it is a journey with stops and detours along the way to examine things off the beaten track, smell the flowers, meet new friends and visit with old friends. - PJM

Life is a bowl of cherries that includes both the pits and the stems. - BAL

Acknowledgements

The authors would like to acknowledge the support of our families (Micky, Heather, Amy and Tim - PJM; Margey - BAL) and our colleagues JAM, BLG and TSD. Deserving of special gratitude for their help and patience are Erica Luper, our secretary, and the editorial staff at Mosby — Jim Shanahan and Jennifer Roche.

We would especially like to acknowledge Barry A. Shapiro, M.D., for his guidance in this endeavor.

Introduction

Arterial blood gases are among the most valuable diagnostic tools available to practitioners of critical care medicine. They are also among the least understood of these tools. The study of acid-base and blood gas physiology is an important facet to the understanding and mastery of pulmonary physiology and pathophysiology.

This workbook is designed to aid in mastery of these topics. While keyed to the first ten chapters of Shapiro's *Clinical Application of Blood Gases*, this workbook can also serve as a stand-alone review text on acid-base and blood gas physiology. The question of why this workbook covers only the first ten chapters of Shapiro has been raised by colleagues and reviewers. The answer is simple: Chapters 1-6 cover the scientific and physiologic basis of ABG and acid-base studies. The remaining chapters (7-10) deal with the appropriate application of acid-base and blood gas data to acute clinical situations. These are the areas which generally cause the new learner studying arterial blood gases the most problems, and these are the areas on which we decided to concentrate.

In large part, the remainder of Shapiro's text (Chapters 11-27) deals with measuring and analytical systems, equipment and techniques of sampling, and quality assurance issues. Additionally, sample case studies are presented in those chapters which allow application of the content of the text.

The workbook is designed to present the concepts, facts and theories covered in Shapiro in several different ways in order to provide a learning tool applicable to varied learning styles. Thus, a content area is often presented using several approaches. We feel that any redundancy is valuable if it allows for fuller comprehension of this difficult subject matter.

Any factual or interpretive errors in this workbook are the fault of the authors and should not and do not reflect on the accuracy of Dr. Shapiro's text. As we end this introduction, we would like to take this opportunity to thank Barry Shapiro, M.D., for his support and trust in this project. Thanks, Barry.

How to use this workbook

The workbook is specifically structured to provide a balance between the attainment of new knowledge and the application of that knowledge. Each chapter has a similar framework designed to lead the learner into a full understanding of Shapiro's text. Generally, the content of each chapter is presented in the following order and format:

Objectives - This section provides learning objectives keyed to the chapter content from both the text and the workbook.

Definitions - This section presents new and/or important words, phrases, and symbols and their meanings.

Introduction - This portion of the chapter summarizes the content of the text chapter, adding some interpretation to the more difficult concepts.

Key Points - This section provides a detailed list of Shapiro's most important statements in the text chapter. These points provide a focus for review and self-assessment.

Tables and Figures - Each chapter of the workbook contains several tables and/or figures, some from the text and some designed especially for the workbook. These tables and figures summarize important information and should be consulted to clarify concepts and information.

Formulas - All formulas presented in the text are duplicated in the workbook. We have also included other useful formulas in the appropriate chapters.

Problems - Each chapter of the workbook contains problems to use as a self-review. We recommend that you treat these questions as a test; do not look at the answers until you complete the practice problems.

Answers to Problems - The answer to each problem in the previous section is provided along with the rationale for that selection.

Application Exercises/Case Studies - This portion of the workbook chapter gives you a chance to test your knowledge with case studies, problem situations and other activities. We have provided solutions for the application exercises/case studies in Chapters 1-3 and Chapter 6. These are not necessarily the only answers but give some insight into our problem solving approach. Chapters 4-5 and 7-10 do not have answers so that the course instructor can apply his or her own methods to the application exercise problems.

Suggested Additional Readings - Each chapter includes a bibliography of additional sources relevant to the topic covered in that chapter. These readings either expand upon the content in Shapiro and this workbook or present the topic in a slightly different way. We urge the reader to consult these excellent sources.

Review Questions - At the end of the workbook there is a self-test which consists of questions from each of the ten chapters of the workbook. These questions are comprehensive and should provide the reader with a challenge. The answers to the review questions are provided in a key following the questions but without explanation.

We suggest that persons utilizing this workbook for review do so in the order that material is presented. Instructors may wish to have their students begin by reviewing the objectives and definitions, followed by the introduction and key points. The tables, figures and formulas will help explain lecture material. Problems and application exercises will be most helpful when used to supplement lecture topics. The review questions provide a comprehensive test bank for the instructor's use.

Contents

CHAPTER 1

Metabolic Acid-Base Balance

Objectives

After reading Chapter 1 and successfully completing this chapter of the workbook the student will be able to:

1. Given the appropriate data, identify the acid-base status of a series of patients.
2. Discuss the concept of ionic dissociation.
3. Define and give examples of dissociation.
4. Define and provide examples of the process of buffering.
5. Write and discuss the chemical equation relating H_2CO_3 production to metabolic end products.
6. Define and compare weak acids and weak bases.
7. Differentiate between volatile and nonvolatile compounds.
8. Define the term *end product.*
9. Write the Henderson-Hasselbalch Equation.
10. Explain the significance of the Henderson-Hasselbalch Equation.
11. Assuming the appropriate data, use the Henderson-Hasselbalch Equation to calculate pH.
12. Discuss why water has a pH of 7.00 in terms of pK_w and the dissociation of H^+ and OH^-.
13. Given the appropriate data, calculate anion gap values.
14. State the pK for human plasma.
15. State the solubility coefficient for CO_2.
16. Define the standard bicarbonate and compare it with CO_2 combining power.
17. Define the following terms/symbols:

acidemia	metabolic alkalosis
alkalemia	metabolite
anion	pH
anion gap acidosis	red cell mass
anion gap anhydrase	respiratory acidosis
carbonic anhydrase	respiratory alkalosis
cation	uncalculated anion
ion	uncalculated cation
metabolic acidosis	[ ]

18. List three therapeutic interventions which may result in increased uncalculated cations.
19. Name three sources of nonvolatile acid metabolites which may cause anion gap acidosis.
20. Name two major sources of hyperchloremic acidosis.

Definitions

acid A substance which will donate hydrogen (H^+) ions to a solution (strong acids donate many H^+ ions; weak acids donate few H^+ ions to the solution).

acidemia pH is more acidic (lower) than normal, below 7.35 (determined by H^+ levels).

acidic solution $[H^+]$ ions outnumber $[OH^-]$ ions. Kw still $= 1 \times 10^{-14}$.

acidosis More acid than bases in the solution (determined by HCO_3^- plasma levels; pH may be within normal range).

aerobic With oxygen or oxygen utilizing.

alkalemia pH is more basic (higher) than normal, above 7.45 (determined by H^+ levels).

alkalosis More base than acid in the solution (determined by HCO_3^- plasma levels; pH may be within normal range).

anaerobic Without oxygen.

anion Negatively (–) charged ions (H^+ acceptors).

anion gap The mathematical difference between the measured cations and the measured anions in the blood plasma.

base A substance which will accept hydrogen (H^+) ions from a solution (strong bases accept many H^+ ions; weak bases accept few H^+ ions from the solution).

base excess/deficit The deviation from the "normal" buffer status. May be either deficit (–) or excess (+).

basic solution $[OH^-]$ ions outnumber $[H^+]$ ions. Kw still $= 1 \times 10^{-14}$.

bicarbonate The HCO_3^- ion, a "weak" base.

buffered A biochemical process through which the effects of strong acids or bases are mediated resulting in a relatively stable and moderate physiologic pH.

[ ] Symbol for "concentration," the amount of solute per unit of solvent.

carbonic acid H_2CO_3, a "weak" acid.

carbonic anhydrase An enzyme which increases the rate of carbonic acid formation by hydrating (adding H^+) and dehydrating (reducing H^+) CO_2.

catalyst A substance which affects the rate of a chemical reaction or changes that reaction's outcomes but is itself not changed or consumed by that reaction.

cation Positively (+) charged ion (H^+ donors).

CO_2 combining power Measured using an anaerobic plasma sample exposed to an equilibrated endtidal air sample.

dissociation The tendency or ability of a substance to break into its constituent elements or into intermediate compounds. Dissociation usually occurs in liquid environments or solutions.

extracellular Outside the cell.

Henderson-Hasselbalch (HH) Equation Mathematical expression of the physiologic acid-base relationship.

homeostasis The tendency of the body to maintain the stability of its chemical, physical and electromechanical systems in a state of dynamic balance. It involves a continuous process of adaptation and change in response to internal and external environmental factors.

hydroxyl ion The OH^- ion.

intercellular Between cells.

intercellular metabolism The physiologic processes of energy production and use within the cells.

intracellular Within the cell.

ion An electrically charged atom or compound. May be either negative (–) or positive (+).

Ka Dissociation constant of an acid (a).

ketoacidosis Increased H^+ due to reduced cellular glucose. Usually secondary to insulin deficiency. Also called diabetic acidosis.

Kw Dissociation constant of H_2O (1×10^{-14}).

logarithm The power to which 10 must be raised to equal a given number.

metabolites (end products) The biochemical elements or compounds which remain after the production of energy through metabolic processes.

mole/L 1 gram equivalent weight of a solute in each liter of solute.

neutral solution A solution whose $[H^+]$ and $[OH^-]$ are nearly equal. pH $\simeq$ 7.00.

nonvolatile substance A substance which does not change state easily (stable).

pathogenic metabolites Metabolic end products which produce effects resulting in a disruption of the body's homeostatic balance.

pH Shorthand notation which describes the **hydrogen ion (H^+) activity** or hydrogen ion concentration in a solution. pH is usually expressed to the second decimal point; e.g., 7.12.

pK pH point at which the solute is 50% dissociated (i.e., the point of maximum buffering capacity).

plasma bicarbonate A HCO_3^- value calculated from plasma pH and PCO_2.

red blood cell mass The total amount of red blood cells in the body.

sodium (Na) pump A biophysical mechanism that redistributes sodium across cell membranes into the extracellular spaces.

solubility coefficient A mathematical constant that reflects the relative ability of a solute to break into its constituent ions in a solvent (to form an ionic solution).

standard bicarbonate Bicarbonate (HCO_3^-) measured in fully oxygenated blood exposed to CO_2 at 40 mmHg pressure at 37° C.

uncalculated cations/anions Electrolytes (ions) measured or unmeasured which are not included in the anion gap calculation.

volatile substance A substance which can change its state or composition.

volatility The relative rate of change of state or composition.

Introduction

In Chapter 1 Shapiro discusses the important concepts of metabolic acid-base balance. In the course of this discussion he not only explains the basics of metabolic acidosis and alkalosis but also covers the following related ideas, mechanisms and equations:

pH – definition and calculation
metabolites – metabolic end products
the carbonic acid cycle
volatile vs. non-volatile acids
buffer systems
Henderson-Hasselbalch Equation – derivation and use
anion gap – function and calculation

Shapiro provides a logical and concise progression of equations detailing the derivation of the Henderson-Hasselbalch (HH) Equation. He first discusses the dissociation constant of water (Kw). Then he derives the HH Equation and its clinical modifications, pointing out its clinical implications. He next discusses the renal compensation (buffering) mechanisms. He describes three methods by which the kidney eliminates H^+ ions. The filtration and carbonic anhydrase production functions of the kidney are also introduced in this chapter. Renal response to acid-base status changes is the next issue considered. Shapiro presents metabolic and respiratory acidosis and alkalosis states, describing the mechanisms by which the kidneys work to mediate acid-base disorders and maintain a dynamic homeostasis. These range from phosphate and ammonia buffer systems in metabolic acidosis to increased H^+ elimination and/or increased HCO_3^- introduction into the blood.

In terms of alkalotic states, HCO_3^- reclamation from the urine is an important defense against metabolic alkalosis. Hypokalemia (decreased plasma K^+) and hyponatremia (reduced plasma Na^+), however, reduce the efficiency of HCO_3^- reclamation from the urine. In respiratory alkalosis, decreased PCO_2 results in a decrease in H^+ production through carbonic anhydrase activity and therefore decreases HCO_3^- retention and reduces H^+ excretion.

The effects of abnormal electrolytes on the renal buffer systems and the hemoglobin buffers can be profound. Potassium (K^+) ions are moved to the extracellular spaces because of the Na^+ pump mechanism. Hemoglobin (Hb) thus exists as a weak acid in equilibrium with its weak K^+ salt (KHb). The K^+ ions can be exchanged for H^+ ions in the distal renal tubules. Reduced Na^+ requires renal reabsorption, thereby deferring HCO_3^- reclamation and H^+ ion excretion. Chloride (Cl^-) ion depletion reduces renal tubule cation exchange in preference to anions such as HCO_3^-.

Shapiro next discusses the concept of anion gap. Anion gap is a calculated value which describes the (charge) inequality between the major cations (K^+, Ca^+, Mg^+) and the major anions (Na^-, Cl^-, HCO_3^-). The "normal" anion gap equals 8-16 mMol/L. He also defines some common sources of anion gap disturbance. These include lactic acidosis, ketoacidosis, acidosis of renal failure and toxic anion gap acidosis. (See Chapter 13 of the text for more details.) Additionally, Shapiro discusses nonanion gap acidosis. This typically occurs with increased Cl^- plasma levels which replace reduced plasma HCO_3^- as in renal tubular acidosis or acute massive diarrhea or chronic diarrhea.

Metabolic acid-base disturbances are indicated by plasma HCO_3^- levels outside of the normal range. Remember that HCO_3^- is part of the Henderson-Hasselbalch Equation. Therefore HCO_3^- can be calculated from measured pH and PCO_2 values obtained through blood gas analysis. Determination of the status of buffering capacity of the blood can be carried out through calculation of the base excess or base deficit. These can be calculated independently of the compensating PCO_2 changes.

Lastly, Shapiro points out the differences between the terms *acidosis* and *alkalosis* and *acidemia* and *alkalemia*.

Key Points

- Life processes require a narrow range of pH.
- Normal metabolism results in the production of end products (metabolites) which form acids in aqueous (water) solutions.
- The major acid-forming metabolite is carbon dioxide (CO_2). 98% of normal metabolite end products are CO_2.
- CO_2 reacts with water (H_2O) to form carbonic acid (H_2CO_3), a volatile acid.
- H_2CO_3 can easily be reconverted to H_2O and CO_2 gas which can be exhaled ($H_2CO_3 \longleftrightarrow H_2O + CO_2$).
- Nonvolatile acids (1-2% of normal metabolites) are buffered.
- Strong acids donate many H^+ ions to the solution; weak acids donate relatively few H^+ ions to the solution.
- Strong bases accept many H^+ ions from the solution; weak bases accept relatively few H^+ ions from the solution.
- H^+ ion concentration ($[H^+]$) is referred to as pH.
- pH ranges from 0 to 14. The pH of pure water is 7.00.
- The ionization constant of water (Kw) is 1×10^{-7}.
- Water dissociates weakly to form H^+ and OH^- ions.
- The $[H^+] = 1 \times 10^{-7}$ ions and $[OH^-] = 1 \times 10^{-7}$ ions.
- Since $[H^+] = [OH^-]$ the solution is considered to be neutral.
- $H^+ + HCO_3^- \longleftrightarrow H_2CO_3 \longleftrightarrow H_2O + CO_2$; the H_2CO_3 cycle can be bi-directional.
- The Henderson-Hasselbalch Equation states:

$$pH = pK + \log\frac{[HCO_3^-]}{[H_2CO_3]} \simeq pH = pK + \log\frac{[HCO_3^-]}{PCO_2}$$

- pH is a ratio of $[HCO_3^-]$ to $[H_2CO_3]$ or $[HCO_3^-]$ to PCO_2.
- pK is 6.1 for human blood.
- The solubility coefficient for CO_2 is 0.0301.
- Normally renal blood flow should lose H^+ ions and gain HCO_3^- ions.
- pH is regulated by the kidney through two mechanisms: active exchange of H^+ and Na^+ ions in the renal glomerular tubules and the production of carbonic anhydrase by renal epithelial cells.
- Carbonic anhydrase is an enzyme (catalyst) which enhances the hydration and dehydration of CO_2.
- The kidney uses three methods to excrete H^+: reabsorption of filtered HCO_3^-, phosphorylation and ammonia formation. All of these cause HCO_3^- and Na^+ to enter the blood while H^+ is eliminated.

- The kidney controls both H^+ excretion in the urine and HCO_3^- reabsorption from the urine.
- Metabolic acid-base balance is dependent on the total amount of H^+ excreted.
- In order for phosphate and ammonia buffers to work in metabolic acidosis, adequate plasma sodium and phosphate levels must be present.
- Due to intercellular K^+ availability, hemoglobin (Hb) exists as a weak acid in equilibrium with the potassium salt (KHb).
- K^+ can be exchanged for H^+ in the distal renal tubule.
- In **respiratory acidosis** rising PCO_2 in the tubular cells causes increased intercellular $[H^+]$ which increases H^+ removal and HCO_3^- addition to the blood.
- Prevention of **metabolic alkalosis** requires normal Na^+ and K^+ plasma levels to reduce HCO_3^- reclamation and thus reduce plasma H^+ levels.
- **Respiratory alkalosis** is characterized by reduced PCO_2 which inhibits the carbonic anhydrase system's ability to both eliminate H^+ through and reclaim HCO_3^- from the urine.
- K^+ ions are primarily distributed to the intercellular spaces by the sodium pump mechanism which forces Na^+ into the extracellular compartment displacing the K^+ ions.
- If the sum of the serum cations (positively charged ions) is subtracted from the sum of the serum anions (negatively charged ions), the remainder is the anion gap. (K^+ is often not included in the calculation.)
- Normal anion gap is 8-16 mMol/L (12-20 mMol/L adding K^+).
- Decreased anion gap is commonly associated with decreased uncalculated anions or, less commonly, with increased uncalculated cations.
- Increased uncalculated cations may occur with Polymyxin-B, calcium or magnesium administration.
- Increases in uncalculated anions will cause anion gap acidosis and may occur secondary to metabolic acidosis, excessive organic salt therapy (Ringer's Lactate, etc.), dehydration or renal failure.
- Decreases in uncalculated cations may also result in anion gap acidosis.
- Anaerobic metabolism causes increased lactic acid and eventual lactic acidosis. This can be reversed by returning to aerobic metabolism.
- Some anaerobic metabolism is normal (in red and white blood cells, the brain and skeletal muscles). (See Chapter 13 of the text for more details.)
- Inability to utilize or produce glucose leads to ketoacidosis and is most often found in diabetics who don't produce insulin. (See Chapter 13 of the text for more details.)
- Renal failure results in retention of both organic and inorganic acids.
- Ingestion of toxic substances can cause anion gap acidosis. Examples include methanol, ethylene glycol and acetic acid.
- Increased plasma Cl^- occurs secondary to loss of plasma HCO_3^- and may be due to diarrhea or renal wasting.
- A key factor in determining metabolic acid-base status is the normality of the plasma HCO_3^-. This can be calculated from the pH and PCO_2.
- CO_2 combining power is measured using an anaerobic plasma sample exposed to an equilibrated endtidal gas sample.
- Standard CO_2 is measured in blood at 100% O_2 and 40 mmHg CO_2 at 37° C.
- Buffering capacity is defined in terms of base excess or base deficit.
- Acidosis and alkalosis refer to whether the acids or the bases are dominant in the plasma.
- Acidemia and alkalemia refer to the pH of the blood.

Tables and Figures

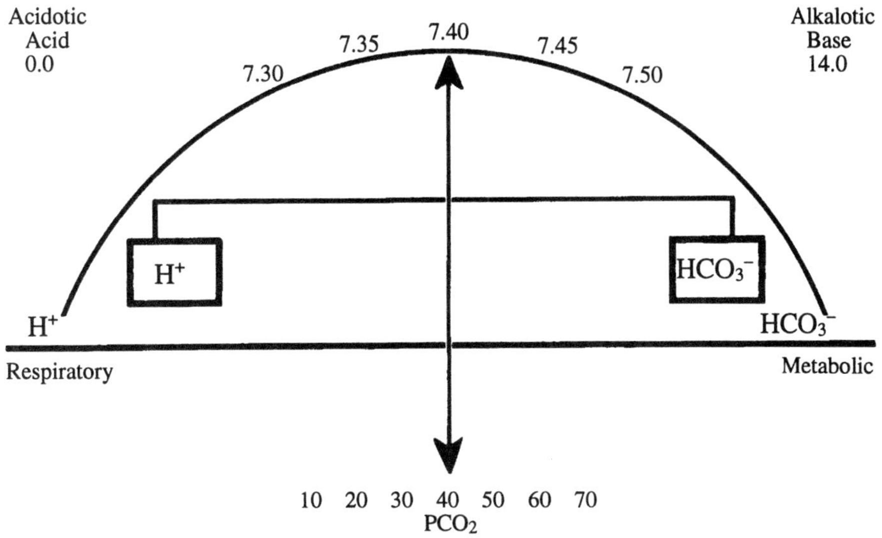

Figure 1: Graphic illustration of an acid-base balance model. As the PCO_2 (H^+ ion concentration) increases, the pH decreases (becomes more acidic). These changes can be balanced by increasing HCO_3^-. Note that normal arterial pH is slightly on the alkalotic side.

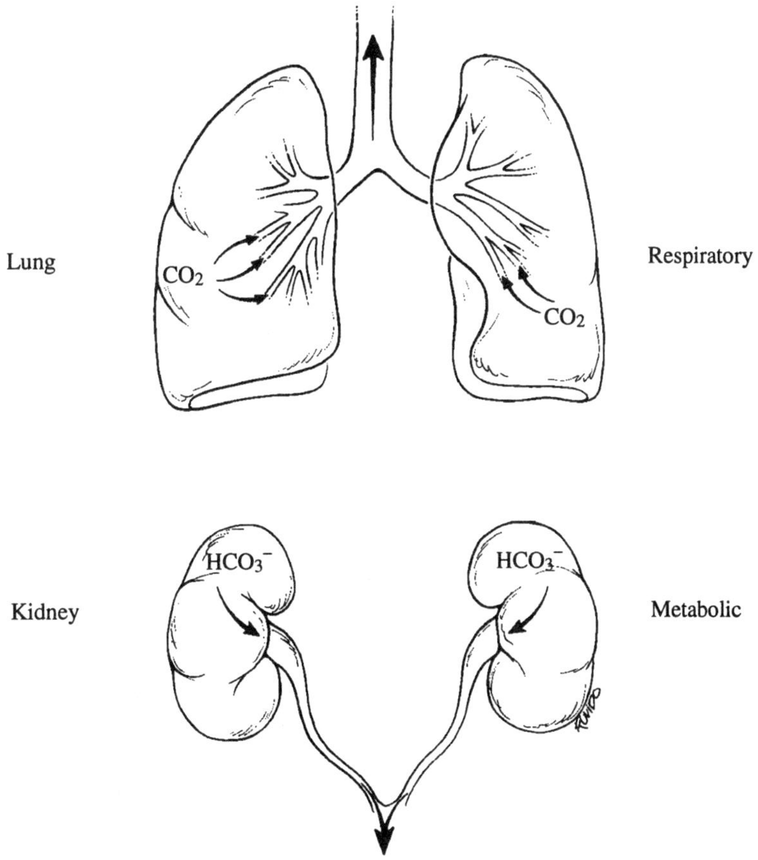

Figure 2: Illustration of the primary functions of the lungs and kidneys in acid-base balance. Note: The kidneys are responsible for metabolic components and the lungs for respiratory components of acid-base balance.

	Units	*Mean*	*Normal* *2 SD* *1 SD*	*Acidotic*	*Alkalotic*
pH	—	7.40	7.35 - 7.45 7.38 - 7.42	< 7.35	> 7.45
PCO_2	mmHg	40	35 - 45 38 - 42	< 45	> 35
HCO_3^-	mMol/L	25	22 - 28 24 - 26	< 22	> 28
			$pH \simeq [HCO_3^-] \mid PCO_2$		

Table 1: Normal values and ranges for serum acid-base indicators. The above table indicates the mean 1 and 2 standard deviation ranges and the decision points for the three main clinical indicators of acid-base status.

Formulas

Carbonic Acid Equilibrium Reaction

$$H_2O + CO_2 \longleftrightarrow H_2CO_3$$

Ionization (Dissociation) Constant of Water (K_{H2O} or Kw)

$$H_2O \longleftrightarrow H^+ + OH^-$$

$$Kw = \frac{[H^+]\ [OH^-]}{H_2O}$$

Modified Kw formula

$$Kw = [H^+]\ [OH^-]$$

$$Kw = [1 \times 10^{-7}]\ [1 \times 10^{-7}]$$

$$Kw = [1 \times 10^{-14}]\ *$$

* The total number of H^+ and OH^- ions in the solution equals 0.00000000000001 liters of H_2O.

Henderson-Hasselbalch (HH) Equation Derivation

$$H_2CO_3 \longleftrightarrow H^+ + HCO_3^-$$

$$Ka = \frac{[H^+] + [HCO_3^-]}{[H_2CO_3]} \text{ but:}$$

$$\text{Log } Ka = \frac{\text{Log } [H^+] + [HCO_3^-]}{[H_2CO_3]}$$

$$\text{Log } Ka = \text{Log } [H^+] + \text{Log} \frac{[HCO_3^-]}{[H_2CO_3]}$$

$$-\text{Log } [H^+] = -\text{Log } Ka + \text{Log} \frac{[HCO_3^-]}{[H_2CO_3]} \text{ but:}$$

$$-\text{Log } [H^+] = pH \text{ and } -\text{Log } Ka = pK = 6.1; \text{ thus:}$$

$$pH = pK + \text{Log} \frac{[HCO_3^-]}{[H_2CO_3]}$$

$$[H_2CO_3] \simeq \text{Sol. Coefficient } PCO_2\ (0.0301) \times PCO_2$$

$$[H_2CO_3] \simeq (0.0301) \times PCO_2; \text{ thus:}$$

$$pH = 6.1 + \text{Log} \frac{[HCO_3^-]}{0.0301 \times PCO_2}$$

Carbonic Acid Formation

$$H_2O + CO_2 \longleftrightarrow H_2CO_3 \overset{CA*}{\longleftrightarrow} HCO_3^- + H^+$$

* carbonic anhydrase enzyme system

Renal pH Buffering Systems

$PCO_2 \longrightarrow CO_2 + H_2O \longrightarrow^{*} HCO_3^- + H^+ +$

a. $HCO_3^- \longrightarrow CO_2 + H_2O$ or
b. $HPO_4 \longrightarrow H_2PO_4-$ or
c. $NH_3 \longrightarrow NH_4-$

* carbonic anhydrase enzyme system

Anion Gap Calculation

Anion Gap = (Major plasma anions) − (Major plasma cations)

$$\text{Anion Gap} = ([Cl^-] + [HCO_3^-]) - [Na^+]$$

or

$$\text{Anion Gap} = ([Cl^-] + [HCO_3^-]) - ([Na^+] + [K^+])$$

Problems

Select and mark the best answer.

1. The Henderson-Hasselbalch Equation essentially quantifies the relationship between ______ and ______ in maintaining acid-base homeostasis.
   a. pH and $[Cl^-]$
   b. kidneys and lungs
   c. pH and P_B
   d. lactic acid and glucose
   e. carbonic anhydrase and NH_3

2. Which of the following formulas is the Henderson-Hasselbalch Equation?
   a. $F_ACO_2 = \frac{\dot{V}CO_2}{\dot{V}_A}$
   b. $P_ACO_2 = \frac{\dot{V}CO_2\ (P_B - 40)}{\dot{V}_A}$
   c. $pH = pK - Log\frac{[HCO_3^-]}{PCO_2\ (0.03)}$
   d. $pH = pK + Log\frac{[HCO_3^-]}{PCO_2\ (0.03)}$
   e. $[HCO_3^-] - [PCO_2] = [pH]$

3. The pK of plasma is
   a. 7.45.
   b. 6.1.
   c. 7.38.
   d. 6.4.
   e. 1×10^{-7}.

4. Given the following data, calculate the anion gap:

	Normal	Measured
	mMol/L	
Na^+	135-145	127
K^+	3.5-5.0	6.8
Cl^-	95-105	98
HCO_3^-	22-26	22

   a. 265.8
   b. 200.2
   c. 149.8
   d. 15.2
   e. 13.8

5. When a large anion gap is reported, the first thing the clinician should do is
   a. reduce K^+ and Cl^- supplements in the patient's diet.
   b. see if K^+ was included in the calculation.
   c. request arterial blood gases to check arterial pH.
   d. suggest increased Na^+ IV or PO intake.
   e. check for increased plasma albumin levels.

6. The anion gap in question 4 is due to
   a. uncalculated cations.
   b. uncalculated anions.
   c. the anion gap is within normal range.
   d. calculated cations.
   e. calculated anions.

7. In nonanion gap metabolic acidosis, chloride [Cl] increases to compensate for
   a. reduced K^+ plasma levels.
   b. increased intracellular Na^+.
   c. extracellular H_2O reserves.
   d. decreased lactic acid production.
   e. depleted plasma $[HCO_3^-]$.

8. Which of the following states is not the result of anaerobic metabolism?
   a. Ketoacidosis
   b. Lactic acidosis
   c. Glycolysis
   d. Diabetic acidosis
   e. a, b and c are correct.

9. Which of the following statements is true regarding carbonic anhydrase?
   a. All of the following statements are correct.
   b. Carbonic anhydrase is produced in the kidneys.
   c. Carbonic anhydrase is a HCO_3^- catalyst.
   d. Carbonic anhydrase catalytic activity partly depends on PCO_2.
   e. Carbonic anhydrase helps conserve plasma bicarbonate and reduce plasma H^+.

10. Which of the following set of values will result in an acidotic pH if used in the HH equation?

	PCO_2	HCO_3^-
a.	47	32
b.	40	26
c.	32	24
d.	43	20
e.	38	23

For questions 11-15 use the paired PCO_2 and HCO_3^- values given to calculate the pH using the Henderson-Hasselbalch Equation (see log table in the appendix of the text).

11. PCO_2 40 mmHg; HCO_3^- 24 mMol/L; pH ______

12. PCO_2 35 mmHg; HCO_3^- 30 mMol/L; pH ______

13. PCO_2 50 mmHg; HCO_3^- 24 mMol/L; pH ______

14. PCO_2 14 mmHg; HCO_3^- 8.4 mMol/L; pH ______

15. PCO_2 65 mmHg; HCO_3^- 38 mMol/L; pH ______

Answers to Problems

1. b: [HCO_3^-] quantifies kidney function and PCO_2 quantifies lung function.

2. d: The Henderson-Hasselbalch Equation allows calculation of pH by examining the logarithmic function of the ratio of [HCO_3^-] and PCO_2. This must yield a positive number and account for the pKa of plasma. Thus, the positive log must be added to the pK.

3. b: The dissociation constant for human blood plasma is 6.1, the pH at which both the H^+ and HCO_3^- ions are 50% dissociated. pK is sometimes referred to as the plasma acid dissociation constant (pKa).

4. a: Anion gap represents the difference between the cations (positively charged ions) and the anions (negatively charged ions). The normal range of the ion gap is 12-20 mMol/L if potassium (K^+) is included or 8-16 mMol/L if K^+ is omitted from the equation.

5. e: Although K^+ may or may not be included in the anion gap calculation, its inclusion should be a matter of policy within the institution. Additionally, this value accounts for only a small portion of the anion gap. Plasma albumin, on the other hand, accounts for up to 50% of the anion gap.

6. c: Normal anion gap ranges from 8-16 mMol/L if K^+ is excluded to 12-20 mMol/L if K^+ is included in the calculation.

7. e: Because there is a direct trade of Cl^- for HCO_3^- (note the signs are the same), the anion gap will remain within normal limits; but because the HCO_3^- is the offsetting buffer for H^+ ions and Cl^-, it is not a good mediator of pH. pH will be shifted toward the acidic range.

8. c: Each of the other choices lists a condition or conditions caused by oxygen free metabolism. Answers a and d are synonyms for the same condition. Answer b refers to the end product of cellular anaerobic metabolism.

9. a: Each of the statements describes a true function or characteristic of carbonic anhydrase, an important renal enzyme (catalyst) for the maintenance of acid-base balance through the elimination of H^+ ions and the conservation of HCO_3^-.

10. d: In order for pH to be acidotic, the PCO_2 must be higher than the normal range (35-45) and the HCO_3^- must be equal to or lower than its normal range (22-28 mMol/L). That is, the ratio of HCO_3^- to ($PCO_2 \times 0.03$) must be greater than 20:1.

11. pH = 7.40: This is a "normal" set of PCO_2 and HCO_3^- values resulting in a "normal" pH. The ratio of HCO_3^- to ($PCO_2 \times 0.03$) is $24/(40 \times 0.03) = 24/1.2 = 20/1$ or 20. The Log of 20 = 1.30.

    pH = pK + 1.3; pH = 6.1 + 1.3; pH = 7.40

12. pH = 7.56: This is an example of an alkalotic pH. The ratio of HCO_3^- to ($PCO_2 \times 0.03$) is $30/(35 \times 0.03) = 30/1.05$; reduced this equals a ratio of $\simeq$ 28.6 / 1. The Log of 28.6 = 1.4564.

    pH = pK + 1.4564; pH = 6.1 + 1.4564; pH = 7.5564; pH $\simeq$ 7.56

13. pH = 7.30: This is an example of an acidotic condition. The ratio of HCO_3^- to ($PCO_2 \times 0.03$) is $24/(50 \times 0.03) = 24/1.5$; reduced this equals 16/1. The Log of 16.0 = 1.2041.

    pH = pK + 1.2041; pH = 6.1 + 1.2041; pH = 7.3041; pH $\simeq$ 7.30

14. pH = 7.40: Even though there are serious abnormalities in the HCO_3^- and PCO_2 as reported, the ratio of HCO_3^- to ($PCO_2 \times 0.03$) is $8.4/(14 \times 0.03) = 8.4/0.42$. This approximates 20/1, resulting in a "normal" pH. The Log of 20 = 1. 3010.

    pH = pK + 1.3010; pH = 6.1 + 1.3010; pH = 7.4010; pH $\simeq$ 7.40

15. pH = 7.39: Again we see a case where severely abnormal [HCO_3^-] and PCO_2 result in a "normal" pH. The

reason is the same; the ratio of $[HCO_3^-]$ and $(PCO_2 \times 0.03)$ remains at about 20/1. $38/(65 \times 0.03) = 38/1.95$. Reduced this equals 19.48/1. The Log of $19.48 \simeq 1.2900$.

$pH = pK + 1.2900$; $pH = 6.1 + 1.2900$; $pH = 7.3900$; $pH \simeq 7.39$

Case Study

Chief Complaint: Mary Timmons, a 67-year-old black female, presented to the ER today with a chief complaint of nausea, vomiting and diarrhea of three days' duration.

Clinical Course: Three days prior to admission the patient attended a regional church meeting that included a pot luck picnic.

Pre-admission day 2: She awoke in the middle of the night with a headache, stomach cramps, nausea, vomiting and diarrhea. She woke her husband, who stated she had fever and chills at that time; her temperature was 102.5° F by oral thermometer. Assuming she would recuperate over the course of the day, she remained in bed and drank fluids and broth.

Pre-admission day 1: The symptoms remained unchanged. To combat the headache and the aches and pains she self-administered 2 (60 gr) buffered ASA tablets Q3-Q4° through the next day. She continued to run a temp (99.4-101.3° F). She would vomit and have attacks of diarrhea every 4-5 hours. She continued to push fluids and continued bed rest.

Admission day: The patient was transported to the ER by her husband, who gave the above history. The patient was admitted to the ER at 1:30 A.M. via wheelchair.

Past Medical History: The patient is a married mother of 3 (ABO 1) with no significant neuro, orthopedic, ob or gyn problems or Hx. Six years ago she was diagnosed as having "mild to moderate" COPD secondary to smoking. No previous history of GI or cardiac problems was elicited during the history taking. EENT: no history except for the need for glasses since age 35.

Social History: 20-year smoking history of 1-1.5 ppd. The patient states she stopped smoking at age forty concurrently with the birth of her first grandchild. The patient denies use of ETOH or nonprescribed drugs. Children and spouse L&W, 5 grandchildren L&W. The patient is a cytotechnology supervisor at this institution and is a civic and church leader.

Physical Exam:

Subjective:

The patient is a slim, febrile and mildly disoriented black female. She is hunched over, clutching her stomach, moaning and grimacing in pain. She appears to be short of breath and breathes in short, shallow, rapid respirations. She is responsive but vague in her answers to questions.

Objective:

Abdomen: Bowel sounds are hyperactive; no rebound tenderness although patient states "the muscles hurt when I vomit."
AP scar noted.

Chest: Slight increase in AP diameter. HS normal with slight tachycardia (98-108 bpm). Decreased expiratory sounds in the bases with a slight expiratory wheeze noted. No rhonchi or rales present. Respiratory rate increased, depth decreased.

HEENT: Neck supple, PERRLA, mouth dry and inflamed

Neuro: non-contributory except as noted

GU: deferred

Vital signs:	T	= 99.5° F oral
	P	= 99 beats per minute
	R	= 28 breaths per minute, shallow
	BP	= 132/90

Laboratory: Among other tests, ABGs were drawn to assess her current status relative to her pre-existing COPD. Additionally, bloods for serum electrolytes were drawn simultaneously. A GI motility test was ordered but deferred as the patient was unable to comply with the conditions for the test. Chest x-rays and an EKG were done.

EKG: Mild tachycardia with U waves and flat T waves noted. Rate is increased, rhythm is WNL, no indications of prior cardiac disease. IMP: mild tachycardia, hypokalemia.

CXR: Air bronchogram is noted, decreased aeration in bases, occasional patchy infiltrates noted in periphery. Diaphragm is mildly flattened, AP diameter is increased. IMP: mild to moderate COPD, ? pneumonic process/aspiration.

ABGs

	Norm	Obs
pH	7.35-7.45	7.52
PCO_2	35-45 mmHg	38
PO_2	80-100 mmHg	82
O_2	sat $\geq$ 95%	90

Chemistry

	Norm	Obs
Na^+	135-145 mMol/L	105
K^+	3.5-5.0 mMol/L	2.8
Ca^+	5.0-10.0 mMol/L	4.0
Cl^-	95-105 mMol/L	110
HCO_3^-	22.0-26.0 mMol/L	30.0
Glucose	0.5-1.5 gm/dL	0.6

Hematology

	Norm	Obs
Hb	12-18 gm/dL	16 gm/dL
Hct	37-52%	60%
RBC	4-6 million/mm3	4-6 million/mm3
WBC	6-10 thousand/mm3	18 thousand/mm3
Osmolality	285-295 mOsm/L	288 mOsm/L

1. What is the probable diagnosis for Mrs. Timmons?

2. What is Mrs. Timmons' acid-base balance status?

3. Explain the effects of Mrs. Timmons' symptoms on her acid-base values.

4. Why are her Hb and Hct elevated? What should be done to rectify this? What might you expect to happen to her "lytes" and acid-base balance due to the treatment of her elevated Hb and "crit"?

5. What is Mrs. Timmons' anion gap? Why is this condition present? What additional treatment is indicated to correct the anion gap?

6. What effect did Mrs. Timmons' COPD have on her current problem? How do you think her admission pH and PCO_2 compare with her usual "normal" pH and PCO_2?

7. Should oxygen be given to treat the tachycardia and low PO_2?

8. What respiratory monitoring or evaluation procedures should be ordered?

9. What effect will Mrs. Timmons' temperature have on CO_2 and production of metabolites?

Answers to Case Study Questions

1. Bacteremia, secondary to food poisoning from contaminated food at the church picnic. The vomiting and diarrhea has compromised an already delicately balanced acid-base status.

2. Mixed metabolic and respiratory alkalosis.

3. The metabolic alkalosis is secondary to "acid dumping" caused by the vomiting and diarrhea which result in the loss of metabolic acids (H^+ donors). The respiratory component is due to the tachypnea (because she is a COPD patient we would expect an elevated P_aCO_2).

4. The nausea, vomiting and diarrhea result in decreased absorption and retention of fluids, thus reducing circulating fluid volumes. As a result of the lower volume of fluid, the solute concentrations increase, although the total amount of solute may decrease or remain the same. The increased temperature (pyrexia) will also promote increased insensible water loss further concentrating the solutes (Hb, Hct and electrolytes).

5. Anion Gap $= ([Cl^-] + [HCO_3^-]) - ([Na^+] + [K^+]) =$
$([110] + [30.0]) - ([105] + [2.8]) =$
$(140) - (107.8) = 32.2$

IV administration of a balanced electrolyte solution and reduction /control of nausea, vomiting and diarrhea are the treatments of choice in Mrs. Timmons' care.

6. Given her COPD, Mrs. Timmons' admission pH and P_aCO_2 were probably radically different from her "normal" pH and P_aCO_2. A COPD patient would have elevated CO_2 levels and a normal or low (more acid) pH. As Mrs. Timmons becomes more fatigued, her respiratory efficiency will decrease and her work of breathing (WOB) will increase, resulting in more CO_2 production. The elevated temperature suggests not only an infective process but also increased metabolic rate. The increased metabolic rate will increase O_2 consumption while concurrently increasing CO_2 and metabolite production.

7. No, Mrs. Timmons' PO_2 is in the low normal range. Additional O_2 is not needed and may increase her risk of respiratory distress as her CO_2 levels are below the hypercapnic response levels. Also, her tachycardia is at the high end of the normal range and will decrease as her temperature decreases. Resolution of the pneumonia, tachypnea and hyperventilation should help address the acid-base and PCO_2 problems.

8. Pulse oximetry and endtidal CO_2 should be monitored, as should ECG and cardiac rate. The first two monitors will reduce the need to perform arterial puncture to obtain arterial blood gases. Additionally, aerosolized bronchodilators and steroids in conjunction with high volume aerosols will liquify and decrease the viscosity of secretions which can then be mobilized by using assisted cough and airway clearance techniques.

9. Increased temperature indicates an increase in metabolic rate. As metabolism increases, to produce energy needed to combat infection, so do its end products (CO_2, heat and other metabolites). The result is an increase in temperature and an increase in PCO_2. The increased temperature (pyrexia) will also promote increased insensible water loss, further concentrating the solutes (Hb, Hct and electrolytes).

Note: Only Chapters 1-3 and 6 will include answers to the Application Exercises/Case Studies. The remaining Applications Exercises/Case Studies will be used by the instructor to augment, lead to or enhance Socratic or discovery method dialogue with the students.

Suggested Additional Readings

Davenport, HW, *The ABCs of Acid Base Balance,* 5th rev. edition, University of Chicago Press, Chicago, IL, 1969.

Des Jardins, T, *Cardiopulmonary Anatomy and Physiology,* 2nd edition, Delmar Publishers, Inc., Albany, NY, 1993.

Emmett, M and Narins, RG, "Clinical uses of the anion gap," *Medicine,* 1977, 56:38-54.

Levitzky, MG, *Pulmonary Physiology,* 3rd edition, McGraw-Hill, Inc., New York, NY, 1991.

Oster, JR, Perez, GO and Masterson, BJ, "Use of the anion gap in clinical medicine," *South Med J*, 1988, 81:229-237.

Scanlan, CL, Spearman, CB and Sheldon, RL, *Egan's Fundamentals of Respiratory Care,* 5th edition, C.V. Mosby, St. Louis, MO, 1990.

CHAPTER 2

Physiology of Respiration

Objectives

After reading Chapter 2 and successfully completing this chapter of the workbook the student will be able to:

1. Use Boyle's law, Charles' Law and Gay-Lussac's Law to calculate changes in a gas's temperature, pressure or volume.
2. Identify the three gas laws: Boyle's Law, Charles' Law and Gay-Lussac's Law.
3. Given a problem involving a change in atmospheric conditions, calculate the new gas partial pressures.
4. Describe Henry's Law and Graham's Law.
5. Given the molecular weight of two gases, calculate which gas diffuses faster.
6. Differentiate between the respiratory exchange ratio and the respiratory quotient.
7. Differentiate between internal, external and cellular respiration.
8. Briefly explain why variations in body position alter distribution of ventilation.
9. Briefly explain why variations in body position and cardiac output alter distribution of perfusion.
10. Differentiate between a deadspace unit, a shunt unit and a silent unit.
11. List and describe the four etiologic categories of tissue hypoxia.
12. Define the term *dysoxia* and briefly discuss the causes.

Definitions

anemic hypoxia The etiologic cause of tissue hypoxia that is secondary to an inadequate amount of hemoglobin to carry oxygen.

BTPS Body temperature and pressure saturated; denoting a volume of gas saturated with water vapor at 37° C and ambient barometric pressure.

circulatory hypoxia The etiologic cause of tissue hypoxia that is secondary to inadequate perfusion.

deadspace Areas of the lung that receive ventilation but do not have accompanying perfusion. This represents a high (infinite) $\dot{V}/\dot{Q}$ ratio.

dynamic equilibrium The condition of balance between varying, shifting and opposing forces that is characteristic of living processes.

dysoxia Abnormal utilization of oxygen at the cellular level.

efficiency of gas exchange The ratio of the actual volume of oxygen and carbon dioxide that diffuses across the lung's alveolar-capillary membrane compared with the potential of the lung to perform gas exchange. The closer the actual diffused gas volume is to the lung's potential diffused gas volume, the greater the lung's efficiency.

Graham's Law The rate of diffusion of a gas through porous membranes varies inversely with the square root of its molecular weight.

gravity-dependent areas of the lung The lung zones where the distribution of both perfusion and ventilation is the greatest. The gravity-dependent areas change according to the individual's body position. In the erect position, dependent lung regions are in the bases. In the supine position, dependent areas are located in the posterior aspects of the lung.

Henry's Law At a given temperature, the amount of gas that can be dissolved in a liquid is proportional to the partial pressure of the gas to which the liquid is exposed.

histotoxic hypoxia The etiologic cause of tissue hypoxia that is secondary to an inability of the cell to use oxygen.

homeostasis The tendency of the body to maintain the stability of its chemical, physical and electromechanical systems in a state of dynamic balance. It involves a continuous process of adaptation and change in response to internal and external environmental factors.

hypoxemic hypoxia The etiologic cause of tissue hypoxia that is secondary to inadequate arterial oxygenation. This type of hypoxia is the result of $\dot{V}/\dot{Q}$ inequality.

partial pressure Pressure exerted by each of the constituents of a mixture of gases.

permeable membrane One permitting the passage of all the substances through the membrane.

pressure gradient A graded difference in the pressure exerted by molecules or ions in a solution or mixture that affects the direction and rate of molecular movement.

respiratory exchange ratio The ratio of the volume of expired carbon dioxide to the volume of oxygen absorbed by the lungs per unit of time.

respiratory quotient The ratio of the volume of produced carbon dioxide to the volume of oxygen consumed by the cells per unit of time.

silent unit Areas of the lung that are not ventilated or perfused.

shunt unit Areas of the lung that are perfused but not ventilated. This represents a zero $\dot{V}/\dot{Q}$ ratio.

Introduction

The physiology of respiration is one of the most important concepts one must master in order to understand the pulmonary system. In Chapter 2, Shapiro discusses gas laws and their relevance to basic concepts of partial pressure, gas diffusion and gas solubility. With these essential principles introduced, he distinguishes between internal and external respiration. The section on external respiration includes a discussion of how efficiency of the pulmonary system is affected by variables that alter the distribution of ventilation and perfusion. Changes in the $\dot{V}/\dot{Q}$ relationship may impact significantly on gas diffusion and thus the patient's arterial blood gases. In the section on internal respiration, Shapiro emphasizes how cellular gas exchange is dependent upon cellular metabolism, regional perfusion and arterial blood gas contents. He includes the final link in the chain—the ability of the cell to use oxygen. If tissue hypoxia exists from whatever cause, this denies the cell the fuel necessary to generate sufficient energy for normal function. Shapiro also introduces the term *dysoxia*, which describes abnormal utilization of oxygen at the tissue level (VO_2) secondary to inadequate oxygen delivery and/or alterations in the way the cell uses oxygen. There are serious diseases or conditions in which dysoxia may exist, such as Adult Respiratory Distress Syndrome, sepsis or the shock syndrome, to name a few.

Key Points

- If the total number of gas molecules is constant, when one of the three variables (volume, temperature, pressure) remains unchanged while another variable changes its value, the third must change in a predictable manner.
- The total pressure of a mixture of gases is equal to the sum of the partial pressures of the separate components.
- The amount of gas that can be dissolved in a liquid is proportional to the partial pressure of the gas to which the liquid is exposed.
- The diffusibility of a gas is inversely proportional to the square root of its molecular weight.
- External respiration is measured by the respiratory exchange ratio (RR). Internal respiration is measured by the respiratory quotient (RQ). Respiratory homeostasis requires that the RR and RQ be equal.
- Normal arterial blood gases do not mean that there is an absence of cardiopulmonary disease. The system may be able to completely compensate and maintain homeostasis.
- Distribution of ventilation is a function of the regional pressure gradients across the lung. Distribution of perfusion within the pulmonary vasculature is primarily dependent upon gravity and cardiac output.
- Zone 1 is the least gravity-dependent area of the lung and therefore has low or absent pulmonary blood flow. Zone 2 is a lung area with varying intermittent blood flow, and it enlarges or shrinks with changes in cardiac output. Zone 3 is a gravity-dependent area with constant pulmonary blood flow, and as with Zone 2 it enlarges or shrinks with changes in cardiac output.
- Because there are regional differences in the distribution of ventilation and perfusion in the lung, lung units have varying $\dot{V}/\dot{Q}$ ratios. The spectrum of the varying $\dot{V}/\dot{Q}$ ratios results in the "normal" $\dot{V}/\dot{Q}$ of the lung.
- Internal respiration is measured by the RQ. It reflects the relationship between oxygen consumption (250 ml/min) and carbon dioxide production (200 ml/min). The normal RQ is 0.8.
- When inadequate tissue perfusion is present, internal respiration is compromised despite adequate pulmonary function.
- There are four types of tissue hypoxia: hypoxemic hypoxia, anemic hypoxia, circulatory hypoxia, and histotoxic hypoxia.
- Cellular oxygenation is impaired by inadequate oxygen delivery and/or alterations in oxygen utilization.

Formulas

Boyle's Law

$$P_1V_1 = P_2V_2$$

Charles' Law

$$\frac{V_1}{T_1} = \frac{V_2}{T_2}$$

Dalton's Law of Partial Pressures

$$P = p_1 + p_2 + p_3 + \ldots$$

Gay-Lussac's Law

$$\frac{P_1}{T_1} = \frac{P_2}{T_2}$$

Graham's Law of Diffusion

$$\frac{r_1}{r_2} = \frac{d_2}{d_1}$$

Respiratory Exchange Ratio (RR)

$$\frac{\text{Volume } CO_2 \text{ excreted}}{\text{Volume } O_2 \text{ uptake}} \text{ or}$$

$$\frac{P_ECO_2}{P_IO_2 \times \frac{P_EN_2}{P_IN_2} - P_EO_2}$$

Respiratory Quotient (RQ)

$$\frac{\text{Volume } CO_2 \text{ produced}}{\text{Volume } O_2 \text{ consumed}}$$

Tables and Figures

Centigrade	*Conversion*	*Kelvin*
0 C	+ 273	273 K
5 C	+ 273	278 K
10 C	+ 273	283 K
15 C	+ 273	288 K
20 C	+ 273	293 K
30 C	+ 273	303 K
35 C	+ 273	308 K
37 C	+ 273	310 K
50 C	+ 273	323 K
75 C	+ 273	348 K
100 C	+ 273	373 K

(Always convert Centigrade to Kelvin when using the gas laws.)

Table 1: Temperature conversion from Centigrade to Kelvin.

Zone	*Pressure Relationship*	*Flow*
1	$P_A > P_a > P_v$	Minimal or absent
2	$P_a > P_A > P_v$	Intermittent
3	$P_a > P_v > P_A$	Constant

Key: P_A - Alveolar Pressure
P_a - Arterial Pressure
P_v - Venous Pressure

Table 2: Three-zone pulmonary perfusion relationship.

Figures 1, 2 and 3 are taken from *Clinical Application of Blood Gases*, 4th edition, by Shapiro, BA, Harrison, RA, Cane, RD, and Templin, R.

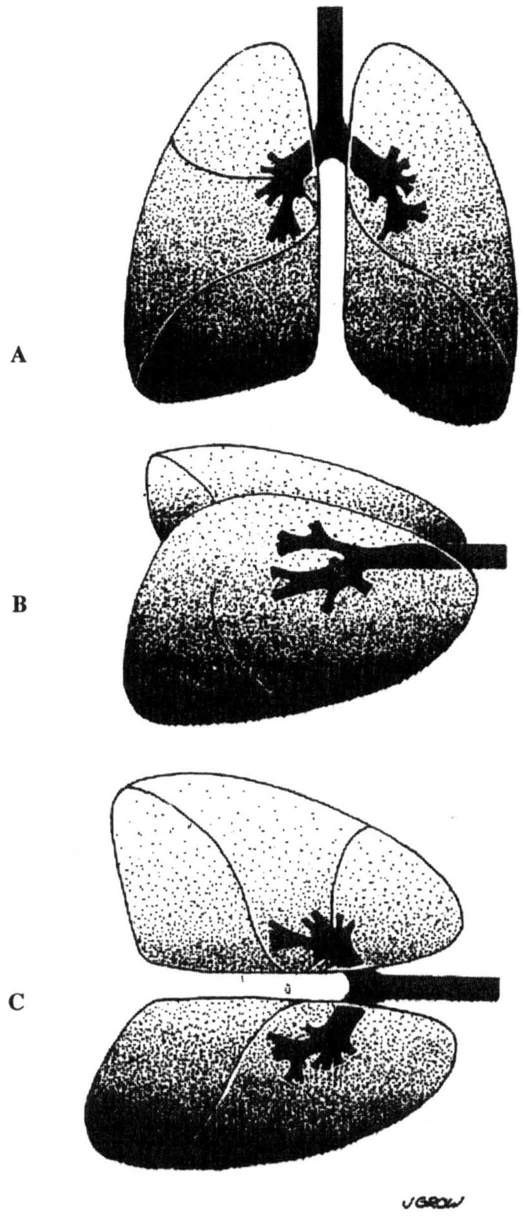

Figure 1: The preponderance of pulmonary blood flow will normally occur in the gravity-dependent areas of the lung. Thus, body position has a significant effect on the distribution of pulmonary blood flow, as shown in the erect (**A**), supine (lying on the back) (**B**), and lateral (lying on the side) (**C**) positions.

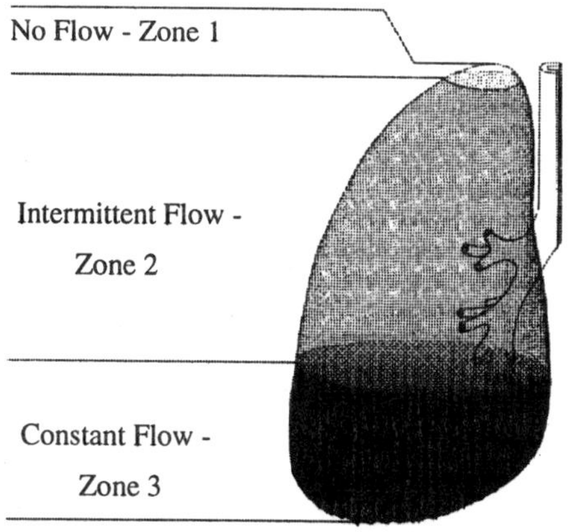

Figure 2: The three-zone model illustrating the effects of gravity on pulmonary perfusion (see text).

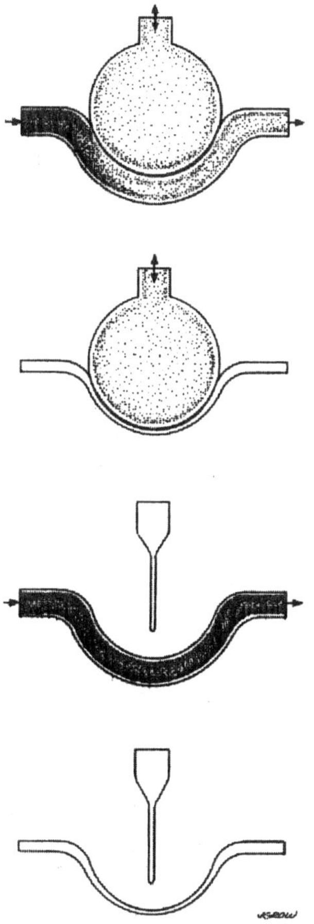

Figure 3: The theoretical respiratory unit. (**A**), normal ventilation, normal perfusion; (**B**), normal ventilation, no perfusion; (**C**), no ventilation, normal perfusion; (**D**), no ventilation, no perfusion.

Problems

Select and mark the best answer.

A sample of gas weighing 0.216 g is trapped in a cylinder by a piston. The volume of the gas is 275 ml when the pressure exerted by the piston is equal to 920 mmHg. If the pressure exerted by the piston is decreased to 780 mmHg, what is the volume? Use this information to answer questions 1-3.

1. What gas law should be used to solve this problem?
   a. Henry's Law
   b. Boyle's Law
   c. Charles' Law
   d. Graham's Law
   e. Gay-Lussac's Law

2. What variable is kept constant in this question?
   a. Time
   b. Volume
   c. Pressure
   d. Temperature

3. What is the new volume in the cylinder?

   ____

4. A low pressure front has moved into the area. Calculate the PO_2 of air with an atmospheric pressure of 720 mmHg. The remaining gases in the atmosphere have the following pressures: pN_2 569 mmHg, PH_2O 20 mmHg, p trace gases 1 mmHg.

   ____

A child's balloon has a volume of 3.80 liters when the temperature is 35° C. What is the volume if the balloon is put into a refrigerator and cooled to 5° C? Assume that the pressure in the balloon is equal to atmospheric pressure at all times. Use this information to answer questions 5-7.

5. What gas law should be used to solve this problem?
   a. Henry's Law
   b. Boyle's Law
   c. Charles' Law
   d. Graham's Law
   e. Gay-Lussac's Law

6. What variable is kept constant in this question?
   a. Time
   b. Volume
   c. Pressure
   d. Temperature

7. What is the new volume in the balloon?

   ____

A steel cylinder of gaseous oxygen has a pressure of 150 atmospheres at a temperature of 20° C. Suppose that the cylinder becomes heated to 75° C because it is stored near a steam radiator. What is the pressure inside the cylinder at the higher temperature? Use this information to answer questions 8-10.

8. What gas law should be used to solve this problem?
   a. Henry's Law
   b. Boyle's Law
   c. Charles' Law
   d. Graham's Law
   e. Gay-Lussac's Law

9. What variable is kept constant in this question?
   a. Time
   b. Volume
   c. Pressure
   d. Temperature

10. What is the new pressure in the cylinder?

    ____

11. At standard conditions 1 liter of oxygen gas weighs approximately 1.44 grams and 1 liter of hydrogen weighs 0.09 grams. Based on the definition of Graham's Law, which gas diffuses faster, oxygen or hydrogen?

    a. ______________________________

    b. How much faster does the gas diffuse?
       a. Two times faster
       b. Three times faster
       c. Four times faster
       d. Five times faster

12. Which of the following equations represents Gay-Lussac's Law?

    a. $P_1V_1 = P_2V_2$

    b. $\frac{V_1}{T_1} = \frac{V_2}{T_2}$

    c. $P = p_1 + p_2 + p_3 + \ldots$

    d. $\frac{P_1}{T_1} = \frac{P_2}{T_2}$

13. Which of the following equations represents Boyle's Law?

    a. $P_1V_1 = P_2V_2$

    b. $\frac{V_1}{T_1} = \frac{V_2}{T_2}$

c. $P = p_1 + p_2 + p_3 + ...$

d. $\frac{P_1}{T_1} = \frac{P_2}{T_2}$

14. What is dysoxia? Describe the possible causes of this oxygenation defect.

____

____

____

15. List and give a brief description of the four etiologic categories of tissue hypoxia and their causes.

a. ______________________________

____

b. ______________________________

____

c. ______________________________

____

d. ______________________________

____

16. Which of the following statements correctly describes a shunt unit within the lung?
    a. It is present in the lungs of normal persons.
    b. It represents that part of the lung perfused by pulmonary capillary blood but not receiving any ventilation.
    c. It represents that part of the lung that is not receiving any capillary blood flow or ventilation.
    d. It is an area of the lung that is receiving ventilation but is not perfused by the pulmonary circulation.
    e. Both a and b are correct.

17. Which of the following statements correctly describes a deadspace unit within the lung?
    a. It results in a low $\dot{V}/\dot{Q}$ in the affected area of the lung.
    b. It represents that part of the lung perfused by pulmonary capillary blood but not receiving any ventilation.
    c. It represents that part of the lung that is not receiving any capillary blood flow or ventilation.
    d. It is an area of the lung that is receiving ventilation but is not perfused by the pulmonary circulation.
    e. Both a and c are correct.

18. What is the effect of the following situations on the distribution of ventilation and perfusion within that individual's lung?
    a. A man changing from a standing position to reclining in bed:

Ventilation distribution

____

____

____

Perfusion distribution

____

____

____

b. An individual who hemorrhaged secondary to a peptic ulcer:

Ventilation distribution

____

____

____

Perfusion distribution

____

____

____

19. State Henry's Law.

____

____

____

20. Show your knowledge of the principles of internal, external and cellular respiration by writing an **ER** next to those items that apply to external respiration, an **IR** next to those that apply to internal respiration and a **CR** next to those that apply to cellular respiration.

_____ a. The diffusion of oxygen across the alveolar-capillary membrane

_____ b. The diffusion of carbon dioxide from the cell into the blood
_____ c. The diffusion of oxygen from the blood into the cell
_____ d. The diffusion of oxygen from the intracellular fluid into the mitochondria of the cell
_____ e. The diffusion of carbon dioxide across the alveolar-capillary membrane into the alveoli to be exhaled
_____ f. The respiratory quotient measures this process
_____ g. The respiratory exchange ratio measures this process
_____ h. The production of ATP within the cell

Answers to Problems

1. b: Boyle's Law

2. d: Temperature

3. 243 ml: V_2
V_2 (new volume) = 275 ml × 920 mmHg/780 mmHg.
In working gas law problems, we are interested in three variable quantities: the volume, the pressure and the temperature. Problem 3 does not mention temperature, therefore we must assume that its initial and final values are the same. We know that pressure is inversely proportional to volume. This means that as pressure decreases, the volume increases. The answer243 ml is consistent with this relationship.

4. $p_B = pN_2 + PH_2O + p_{TG} + PO_2$

$p_B - (pN_2 + PH_2O + p_{TG}) = PO_2$

130 mmHg = 720 − (569 mmHg + 20 mmHg + 1 mmHg)

This question asks you to use the principle of Dalton's Law of Partial Pressures to arrive at the correct answer. The barometric pressure represents the total pressure. The small p's are the individual gases within the atmosphere. Oxygen is the one gas that changes with alterations in the barometric pressure. Water vapor pressure remains the same unless the atmospheric temperature or relative humidity changes. Nitrogen gas is inert and remains constant, and trace gases have no appreciable effect on the total pressure.

5. c: Charles' Law

6. c: Pressure

7. $\frac{V_1}{T_1} = \frac{V_2}{T_2}$ or it may be expressed as:

V_2 (new volume) $= \frac{V_1}{T_1} \times T_2$

$V_2 = \frac{3.80\text{ L}}{308\text{ K}} \times 278\text{K}$

$3.43\text{ L} = V_2$

Charles' Law is the guide in answering this problem. According to this law, when the temperature decreases, the volume must decrease proportionately. Because we can use only absolute temperatures in gas-law calculations, other scales of temperature must be converted to the Kelvin scale: C + 273 = K.

8. e: Gay-Lussac's Law

9. b: Volume

10. $\frac{P_1}{T_1} = \frac{P_2}{T_2}$ or it may be expressed as:

P_2 (new pressure) $= \frac{P_1}{T_1} \times T_2$

$P_2 = \frac{150\text{ atm}}{293\text{ K}} \times 348\text{ K}$

$178\text{ atm} = P_2$

Gay-Lussac's Law is the guide in answering this problem. According to this law, when the temperature increases, the gas molecules move in the cylinder more rapidly, hitting one another and the cylinder walls more often and with greater force. As a result, the pressure increases. The gas is stored in a steel cylinder and its volume does not change. The two variables are temperature and pressure.

11. $\frac{r_1}{r_2} = \frac{d_2}{d_1}$
a. Hydrogen: According to Graham's Law, the rates of diffusion are related to the square roots of their densities. Therefore, it is logical to assume the hydrogen will diffuse faster because it is less dense.
b. c: $r_{H2} = r_{O2} \times$ 1.44 g/liter / 0.09 g/liter
$r_{H2} = r_{O2} \times 1.2 / 0.3 = 4\, r_{O2}$

12. d: Gay-Lussac's Law

13. a: Boyle's Law

14. *Dysoxia* is a term identified by Shapiro to characterize abnormal utilization of oxygen at the cellular level. Dysoxia represents the problem of inadequate delivery of oxygen to the tissues and a defect in the ability of the cell to use the oxygen.

15. Hypoxemic hypoxia: This etiologic category of tissue hypoxia is secondary to inadequate arterial oxygenation

(hypoxemia). It is usually secondary to inadequate respiratory function.

Anemic hypoxia: This etiologic category of tissue hypoxia is secondary to inadequate oxygen carrying capacity. This is usually caused by anemia, hence the name; but it may also occur when the hemoglobin is unable to carry oxygen, as in carbon monoxide poisoning or methemoglobemia.

Circulatory hypoxia: This etiologic category of tissue hypoxia is secondary to inadequate perfusion of the cells. This may be caused by inadequate heart function or abnormal distribution of blood at the tissue level (e.g., a-v shunting).

Histotoxic hypoxia: This etiologic category of tissue hypoxia is secondary to the inability of the cells to use oxygen. The classic example always mentioned as a cause of histotoxic hypoxia is cyanide poisoning.

16. e: A shunt unit is an area of the lung that is perfused by the pulmonary capillary but is completely unventilated. The normal lung contains the spectrum of ventilation/perfusion relationships within the lung. Therefore the normal lung contains deadspace, shunt and silent units.

17. d: A deadspace unit is an area of the lung that is normally ventilated but there is no blood flow. Deadspace results in an increasing (theoretically infinite) ventilation/perfusion ratio. A shunt unit results in a decreasing (theoretically zero) ventilation/perfusion ratio.

18. a. Changing from a sitting to a reclining position: The **distribution of ventilation** changes when an individual moves from a sitting to a supine position. In the erect or sitting position, a greater proportion of the individual's tidal volume goes to the bases of the lung (Zone 3). In the newly assumed reclining position, most of the individual's tidal breath will go to the posterior (dependent) aspects of the lung. This is because the transpulmonary pressure changes are now the greatest in the posterior. Therefore, the ventilation will preferentially distribute to these areas. The **distribution of perfusion** changes when an individual moves from a sitting to a supine position. In the erect or sitting position, a greater proportion of the individual's pulmonary blood flow will distribute to the gravity-dependent areas of the lung, which are in this case the bases of the lung. In the newly assumed reclining position, the posterior aspects of the lung are now the most gravity-dependent areas of the lung. The effect of gravity on the pulmonary arterial pressures results in preferential blood flow through these gravity-dependent regions.

b. Acute hemorrhage secondary to a peptic ulcer: The **distribution of ventilation** does not change in the event of acute hemorrhage. The distribution of lung volume is based on the transpulmonary pressure changes across the lung, and this will not change in this situation.
The **distribution of perfusion** changes when an individual loses blood volume. The effects of gravity on pulmonary perfusion are described in the three-zone model. The lung is divided into three perfusion zones according to the relationship between alveolar, pulmonary arterial and pulmonary venous pressures. Theoretically, Zone 1 has no blood flow, Zone 2 has intermittent blood flow and Zone 3 has continuous flow. Gravity, however, is not the only determinant of pulmonary perfusion. The three perfusion zones are also affected by cardiac output. An acute hemorrhage will decrease cardiac output and decrease blood flow through the pulmonary vasculature. The reduction in blood flow decreases the arterial and venous pressure and changes the distribution of perfusion to the lung. Therefore, in the normal lung, as cardiac output decreases, Zone 3 becomes smaller and Zones 1 and 2 become larger. This will affect the entire lung's $\dot{V}/\dot{Q}$.

19. The quantity of a slightly soluble gas that dissolves in a liquid at a given temperature is directly proportional to the partial pressure of that gas in the gas phase.

20. a. ER b. IR c. IR d. CR e. ER f. IR g. ER h. CR
Gas exchange between the environment (alveoli) and the pulmonary capillary blood is called **external respiration.** Items a, e, g describe the process of the movement of gas across the alveolar capillary membrane. Gas exchange of oxygen and carbon dioxide between systemic capillary blood and the cell is known as **internal respiration.** Items b, c, f describe this process. **Cellular respiration** is the process that includes movement of oxygen into the mitochondria of the cell and the generation of ATP through cellular metabolic pathways. Items d and h describe this essential cellular function.

Application Exercises

Situation 1

The early method of diving by breath holding is still used today to retrieve pearls and sponges from the sea. The breath holding time is usually confined to 60-75 seconds. The individual generally hyperventilates or breathes oxygen prior to descent in order to prolong diving time.

Diver's parameters at water surface:
- Lung volume 6 liters
- Pressure 1 atmosphere (atm)
- BTPS conditions

Diver descends to 3 atmospheres (2 atm caused by the weight of the water and 1 atm by the air above the water). With your knowledge of gas laws, answer the following questions concerning the changes during a breath holding dive:

1. What is the volume within the lungs at the 3 atm depth?

2. What gas law should be used to solve this problem?

3. What are possible physiologic effects of this lung volume change?

Situation 2

You are working in the pulmonary outpatient clinic checking an asthmatic patient's MDI technique when you are told by the patient that he has just taken his first scuba diving lesson. He is very excited about this new recreational activity, and he reassures you that he is a very good swimmer and is physically capable of scuba diving.

1. Using your knowledge of Boyle's Law and asthma, what problems could this man encounter during a scuba dive?

2. Are there any techniques that he could use to prevent the problems associated with asthma and diving?

Answers to Application Exercises

Situation 1

1. $P_1V_1 = P_2V_2$
   $1 \text{ atm} \times 6L = 3 \text{ atm} \times x$
   $6 \text{ L/atm} / 3 \text{ atm} = x$
   $2L = x$

2. Boyle's Law

3. The individual's lung volume is reduced to below the functional residual capacity. Because of the reduction in pulmonary reserve, this might interfere with oxygenation of the arterial blood.

Situation 2

1. There is a risk of air trapping and air embolism in divers with active asthma. Based upon Boyle's Law, the pressure changes that occur with submersion in water coupled with an asthmatic's inability to empty the lungs of air at a normal rate poses a definite risk of lung overexpansion and barotrauma. Diving articles indicate that the greatest danger to asthmatic divers upon ascension is within ten feet of the surface because the fractional pressure changes with depth are the greatest. Therefore, even shallow diving poses a risk for an asthmatic. Most medical consultants consider asthma a contraindication to diving.

2. If an asthmatic still insisted on diving, he/she could optmize lung function before diving. Using the MDI just before diving would improve airflow distribution and lessen the risk of lung overdistention and barotrauma.

Suggested Additional Readings

Kacmarek, RM, Mack, CW and Dimas, S, *The Essentials of Respiratory Care,* 3rd edition, C.V. Mosby, St. Louis, MO, 1990, Chapters 2, 4 and 13.

Scanlan, CL, Spearman, CB and Sheldon, RL, *Egan's Fundamentals of Respiratory Care,* 5th edition, C.V. Mosby, St. Louis, MO, 1990, Chapter 4.

Shapiro, BA, Kacmarek, RM, Cane, RD, Peruzzi, WT and Hauptman, D, *Clinical Application of Respiratory Care,* 4th edition, Mosby-Year Book, St. Louis, MO, 1991, Chapters 7 and 14.

CHAPTER 3

Respiratory Acid-Base Balance

Objectives

After reading Chapter 3 and successfully completing this chapter of the workbook the student will be able to:

1. Given the appropriate data, identify the acid-base state of a series of patients.
2. Identify the ways in which CO_2 is carried within the blood.
3. Identify what percentage CO_2 is carried by the various physiologic mechanisms within the blood.
4. Explain how the mechanisms that carry CO_2 result in very little change in plasma pH.
5. Describe the chloride shift and its role in CO_2 transport.
6. Identify the clinical measurement that reflects respiratory acid-base balance.
7. Describe how changes in alveolar ventilation, alveolar perfusion and mixed venous CO_2 content affect the patient's alveolar CO_2.
8. Identify the equations that allow calculation of:
   a. alveolar ventilation
   b. deadspace ventilation
   c. anatomic deadspace
9. Given the appropriate information, calculate the patient's:
   a. alveolar ventilation
   b. deadspace ventilation
   c. anatomic deadspace
10. Describe the relationship between alveolar ventilation and P_aCO_2.
11. Describe the relationship between deadspace ventilation and respiratory rate.
12. Identify the classification criteria for each of the following respiratory acidic conditions:
    a. uncompensated (acute)
    b. partially compensated (subacute)
    c. compensated (chronic)
13. Identify the classification criteria for each of the following respiratory alkalotic conditions:
    a. uncompensated (acute)
    b. partially compensated (subacute)
    c. compensated (chronic)

Definitions

alveolar deadspace (V_{Dalv}) An alveolus that is ventilated but not perfused. This gas volume reaches the alveoli but does not participate in gas exchange. Normal individuals do not have significant true alveolar deadspace because even the apical segments of the lung receive a small amount of perfusion.

anatomic deadspace (V_{Danat}) The gas remaining in the airway conducting structures at the end of each breath. This gas volume never reaches the alveoli and never participates in gas exchange. It approximates 1 ml/lb of ideal body weight.

buffering mechanisms Applied to the blood, buffering mechanisms are bicarbonate, protein, phosphate and ammonia. These mechanisms are the body's first line of defense against abrupt changes in blood pH. They minimize alterations in pH if a strong acid or base is added to the body.

chloride shift The exchange of bicarbonate anions for chloride anions across the red blood cell membrane. The bicarbonate anions diffuse into the plasma from the RBC and the chloride anions diffuse into the RBC from the plasma. This shift is also known as the "hamburger phenomenon."

compensation The counterbalancing of any defect of structure or function. In acid-base abnormalities, compensation is the process that attempts to restore the blood pH to normal. In respiratory acid-base disorders, compensation occurs through the renal system.

high $\dot{V}/\dot{Q}$ Gas exchange in the alveolus that is in excess of perfusion to the alveolus. This may be due to increased ventilation or decreased perfusion. High $\dot{V}/\dot{Q}$ does not usually represent true alveolar deadspace but is referred to as "relative" alveolar deadspace.

hydrating reaction of carbon dioxide The reaction of carbon dioxide with water to form carbonic acid. This is sometimes called the "hydrolysis reaction" because water is broken down as it reacts with CO_2 to form H_2CO_3.

reduced hemoglobin Unoxygenated hemoglobin.

respiratory acidosis Acidosis resulting from ventilatory impairment and subsequent retention of CO_2 leading to an accumulation of H^+ concentration.

respiratory alkalosis Alkalosis resulting from reduced carbon dioxide tension in the blood caused by hyperventilation leading to a reduced H^+ concentration.

Introduction

In Chapter 3, Shapiro discusses the important concepts of respiratory acid-base balance. In the course of this discussion he explains not only the essential elements of respiratory acidosis and alkalosis but also the concepts that are necessary to understand ventilation and its effect on arterial PCO_2 and acid-base balance.

As an introduction to the concept of respiratory acid-base balance, Shapiro discusses carbon dioxide transport. He briefly discusses the three mechanisms by which carbon dioxide is carried by the blood. First, as with O_2, CO_2 is able to dissolve in the plasma. Five percent of the carbon dioxide is carried in this fashion; but this amount, although small, fluctuates directly with the patient's PCO_2. Carbon dioxide is also carried in chemical combination with amino acids contained within the hemoglobin and the plasma. It is estimated that there is a 20-30% percent increase in the blood's CO_2 transport capabilities when hemoglobin is in the reduced state and carbon dioxide is carried as carbamino compounds. Bicarbonate ion is the third and most important way that CO_2 is carried in the blood. When CO_2 enters the red blood cell, it dissociates into H^+ and HCO_3^-. The hydrogen is buffered by the red blood cell and the bicarbonate diffuses into the plasma. Plasma chloride then diffuses into the red blood cell in order to maintain anion balance. This process is known as the chloride shift.

After the discussion of carbon dioxide transport, the topic of alveolar carbon dioxide follows naturally. Shapiro explains how alveolar ventilation, alveolar perfusion and mixed venous CO_2 content affect the patient's alveolar carbon dioxide partial pressure.

A critical point to remember is that alveolar PCO_2 varies inversely with alveolar ventilation. Shapiro emphasizes that this is key to understanding respiratory acid-base balance. Variations in deadspace can have a large impact on alveolar ventilation. There are two categories of deadspace: anatomic deadspace and alveolar deadspace. Normally, anatomic deadspace is equivalent to normal body weight in pounds. Alveolar deadspace is usually not clinically significant, but diseases or conditions that change the patient's $\dot{V}/\dot{Q}$ will increase the alveolar deadspace.

The discussion of alveolar ventilation continues with a brief discourse on the effect that ventilatory pattern has on deadspace ventilation. Anatomic deadspace impacts less on alveolar ventilation when the tidal volume is larger and when the respiratory rate is slower. If the individual's respiratory rate is fast and/or tidal volume decreases, anatomic deadspace assumes a greater portion of the patient's minute ventilation, which affects alveolar PCO_2. If a disease process is superimposed on the situation, observation of respiratory rate and tidal volume may not be accurate in predicting the adequacy of the patient's ventilation.

The second physiologic parameter affecting alveolar carbon dioxide is alveolar perfusion. Shapiro states that CO_2 diffusion into the alveoli is partly dependent on pulmonary capillary blood flow. If blood flow is low or absent, CO_2 gas exchange is proportionately reduced and alveolar CO_2 levels remain low. If minute ventilation remains the same, this increase in deadspace will decrease alveolar ventilation. Conversely, if pulmonary capillary blood flow returns to normal, deadspace ventilation decreases proportionately, and alveolar ventilation increases and maintains a stable alveolar PCO_2.

Mixed venous CO_2 content is the last important physiologic parameter Shapiro identifies that directly affects alveolar PCO_2 partial pressure. The mixed venous content is the reservoir for diffusion of CO_2 into the alveolus. An elevated CO_2 content stimulates the central respiratory drive which increases alveolar ventilation, thereby attempting to maintain a stable CO_2. If CO_2 content is low, respiratory drive is reduced and therefore alveolar ventilation decreases in an attempt to keep the PCO_2 from fluctuating.

The very important final part of Shapiro's discussion on respiratory acid-base balance is the specification of the criteria used to identify respiratory acidosis and alkalosis. The criteria categories are the patient's pH, PCO_2, plasma bicarbonate and base excess. There are three ways to classify a respiratory abnormality: acute, or uncompensated; subacute, or partially compensated; and chronic, or compensated.

If the condition is acute or uncompensated, the renal system (represented by bicarbonate or base excess) has not started to compensate for the CO_2 loss or gain. In this situation the bicarbonate and base excess are normal and the pH is abnormal.

If the condition is subacute or partially compensated, the renal system has started to compensate; therefore, the bicarbonate and base excess are either elevated or decreased depending upon the acid-base state. Despite these compensatory efforts by the kidney, however, the pH is not within normal range.

Finally, if the condition is chronic or compensated, the respiratory acid-base abnormality has persisted and the renal system has had time to reabsorb sufficient bicarbonate to normalize the pH. In this situation the bicarbonate and base excess are elevated or decreased depending upon the acid-base state, and the pH is within the normal range.

Key Points

➢ Carbon dioxide is transported in the blood in three forms: dissolved in the plasma, in chemical combination with amino acids (carbamino compounds and hemoglobin) and as bicarbonate.

- Carbamino hemoglobin and bicarbonate ion mechanisms allow for a large amount of CO_2 to be transported with little change in H^+ concentration.
- The solubility coefficient and the partial pressure of carbon dioxide determines the amount of CO_2 physically dissolved in solution. Approximately 5% of the CO_2 is carried dissolved in the plasma.
- 20-30% of the carbon dioxide carried in the blood is carried on the globin portion of the hemoglobin molecule. This is a carbamino compound.
- 65-75% of the carbon dioxide that is carried in the blood is in the form of bicarbonate ion.
- The arterial PCO_2 is the essential clinical measurement reflecting the respiratory acid-base balance.
- Alveolar ventilation is the portion of ventilation that participates in gas exchange.
- The alveolar PCO_2 is the result of the interplay among three variables: alveolar ventilation, alveolar perfusion and mixed venous CO_2 content.
- Alveolar ventilation is the sum of alveolar ventilation and deadspace ventilation.
- Alveolar PCO_2 is inversely proportional to alveolar ventilation, and alveolar PO_2 is directly proportional to alveolar ventilation.
- Deadspace ventilation is the result of three physiologic variables: anatomic deadspace, alveolar deadspace and high $\dot{V}/\dot{Q}$ ratio.
- Anatomic deadspace is affected by the patient's ventilatory pattern. The higher the respiratory rate, the greater the deadspace ventilation. The larger the tidal volume, the less effect anatomic deadspace has on alveolar ventilation and alveolar gas tensions.
- Alveolar deadspace is the result of diseases or conditions that increase the patient's $\dot{V}/\dot{Q}$ ratio.
- If alveolar perfusion increases, alveolar ventilation must increase to maintain a stable alveolar PCO_2. If alveolar perfusion decreases, alveolar ventilation must decrease to maintain a stable alveolar PCO_2.
- Mixed venous CO_2 content is the reservoir for CO_2 diffusion from the pulmonary capillary into the alveolus.
- If a patient's mixed venous CO_2 content is increased, the patient's alveolar ventilation must increase in order to maintain a stable alveolar PCO_2. If alveolar ventilation does not change, the alveolar PCO_2 and arterial PCO_2 will increase.
- If a patient's mixed venous CO_2 content is decreased, the patient's alveolar ventilation must decrease in order to maintain a stable alveolar PCO_2. If alveolar ventilation does not change, the alveolar PCO_2 and arterial PCO_2 will decrease.
- The interrelationships of pulmonary and renal responses to acid-base imbalances are predictable.
- A patient with uncompensated respiratory acidosis has a low pH, a high P_aCO_2, and a normal bicarbonate and base excess. This is an acute condition.
- A patient with partially compensated respiratory acidosis has a low pH, a high P_aCO_2, and an increased bicarbonate and positive base excess. This is a subacute condition.
- A patient with compensated respiratory acidosis has a pH within the normal range, an elevated P_aCO_2, and an increased bicarbonate and positive base excess. This is a chronic condition.
- A patient with uncompensated respiratory alkalosis has a high pH, a low P_aCO_2, and a normal bicarbonate and base excess. This is an acute condition.
- A patient with partially compensated respiratory alkalosis has a high pH, a low P_aCO_2, and a decreased bicarbonate and negative base excess. This is a subacute condition.
- A patient with compensated respiratory alkalosis has a a pH within the normal range, a low P_aCO_2, and a decreased bicarbonate and negative base excess. This is a chronic condition.

Tables and Figures

Nomenclature	***pH***	***PCO_2***	***$[HCO_3^-]p$***	***BE***
		Respiratory acidosis		
Uncompensated (acute)	↓	↑	N	N
Partially compensated (subacute)	↓	↑	↑	↑
Compensated (chronic)	N	↑	↑	↑
		Respiratory alkalosis		
Uncompensated (acute)	↑	↓	N	N
Partially compensated (subacute)	↑	↓	↓	↓
Compensated (chronic)	N	↓	↓	↓

Note: Arrows indicate depressed or elevated levels; N is normal; and BE is base excess

Table 1: Traditional respiratory acid-base nomenclature. As shown on page 46 (Table 4-1) in *Clinical Application of Blood Gases,* 4th edition, by Shapiro, BA, Harrison, RA, Cane, RD, and Templin, R.

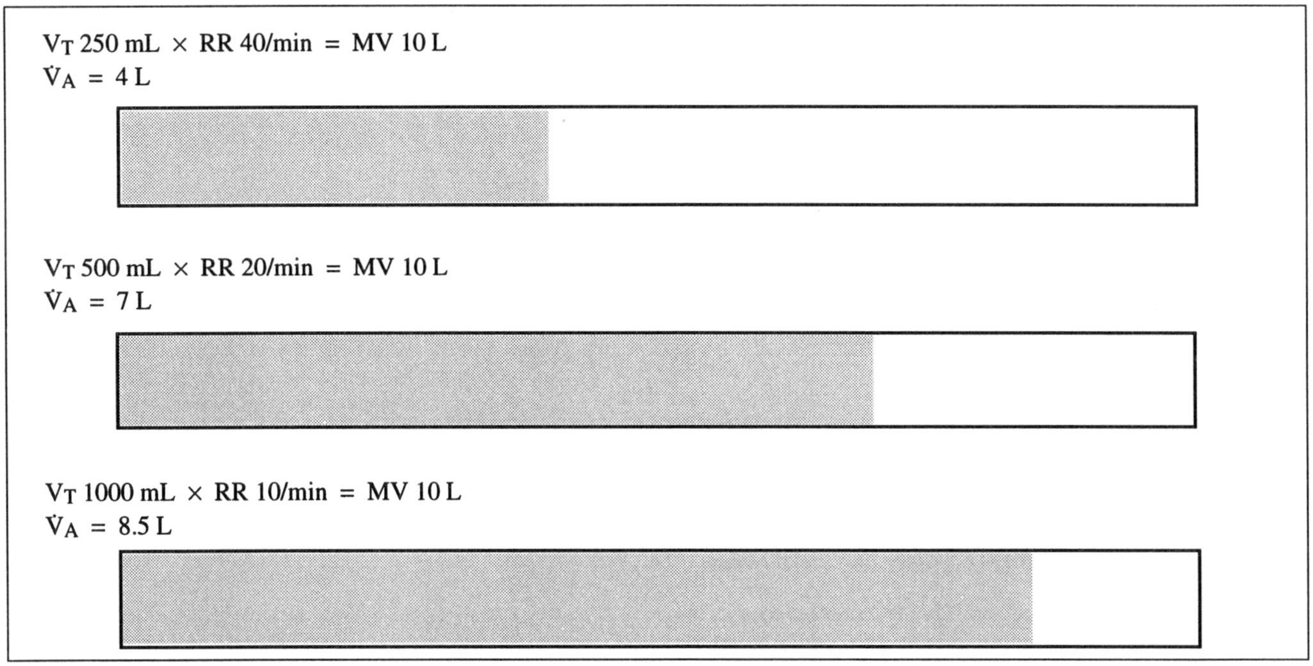

Figure 1: The ventilatory pattern and alveolar ventilation. In all three examples, the minute ventilation (MV) is 10 L. Assuming an anatomic deadspace of 150 ml, the alveolar ventilation ($\dot{V}_A$) varies markedly with changes in ventilatory pattern (V_T = tidal volume, RR = respiratory rate). Obviously, disease can add deadspaces other than the anatomic ones and can cause even greater variances in alveolar ventilation. As shown on page 44 (Figure 4-3) in *Clinical Application of Blood Gases*, 4th edition, by Shapiro, BA, Harrison, RA, Cane, RD, and Templin, R.

Formulas

Anatomic Deadspace

1 ml/lb of ideal body weight
2.2 ml/kg of ideal body weight

Alveolar Ventilation ($\dot{V}_A$)

$$\dot{V}_A = \dot{V}_E - \dot{V}_D$$

Deadspace Ventilation ($\dot{V}_D$)

$$\dot{V}_D = \dot{V}_E - \dot{V}_A$$

Minute Ventilation ($\dot{V}_E$)

$$\dot{V}_E = RR \times V_T \quad \text{or} \quad \dot{V}_E = \dot{V}_A + \dot{V}_D$$

Respiratory Acidosis

$$\uparrow CO_2 + H_2O \overset{CA^*}{\longleftrightarrow} \uparrow H_2CO_3 \longleftrightarrow \uparrow H^+ + \uparrow HCO_3^-$$

(hypoventilation)

* carbonic anhydrase enzyme system

Acute respiratory acidosis
$pH < 7.35 = \uparrow PCO_2 \; / \longleftrightarrow HCO_3^-$

Partially compensated respiratory acidosis
$pH < 7.35 = \uparrow PCO_2 \; / \uparrow HCO_3^-$

Compensated respiratory acidosis
$pH\ 7.35 - 7.4 = \uparrow PCO_2 \; / \uparrow HCO_3^-$

Respiratory Alkalosis

$$\downarrow CO_2 + H_2O \overset{CA^*}{\longleftrightarrow} \downarrow H_2CO_3 \longleftrightarrow \downarrow H^+ + \downarrow HCO_3^-$$

(hyperventilation)

* carbonic anhydrase enzyme system

Acute respiratory alkalosis
$pH > 7.45 = \downarrow PCO_2 \; / \longleftrightarrow HCO_3^-$

Partially compensated respiratory alkalosis
$pH > 7.45 = \downarrow PCO_2 \; / \downarrow HCO_3^-$

Compensated respiratory alkalosis
$pH\ 7.4 - 7.45 = \downarrow PCO_2 \; / \downarrow HCO_3^-$

Problems

Select and mark the best answer.

1. Place a check next to those statements describing the body's biochemical mechanisms that permit the transport of CO_2.
   _____ a. Carried as carbon monoxide
   _____ b. Carried as bicarbonate ion
   _____ c. Carried as carbonic anhydrase
   _____ d. Carried on reduced hemoglobin
   _____ e. Carried as blood urea nitrogen
   _____ f. Carried as carbamino compounds
   _____ g. Physically dissolved in the plasma

2. Which of the following clinical measurements reflects respiratory acid-base balance?
   a. Arterial pH
   b. Arterial PCO_2
   c. Alveolar deadspace
   d. Minute ventilation

3. If the patient's mixed venous CO_2 content increases with no change in alveolar ventilation or alveolar perfusion, what is the effect on alveolar PCO_2?
   a. Increases
   b. Decreases
   c. No change

4. If alveolar perfusion decreases with no change in alveolar ventilation and mixed venous CO_2 content, what is the effect on alveolar PCO_2?
   a. Increases
   b. Decreases
   c. No change

5. Which of the following equations could be used to determine deadspace ventilation?
   a. $\dot{V}_E - \dot{V}_D$
   b. $\dot{V}_E - \dot{V}_A$
   c. $RR \times V_T$
   d. $\dot{V}_A + \dot{V}_D$

6. Which of the following equations could be used to determine alveolar ventilation?
   a. $\dot{V}_E - \dot{V}_D$
   b. $\dot{V}_E - \dot{V}_A$
   c. $RR \times V_T$
   d. $\dot{V}_A + \dot{V}_D$

7. Which of the following equations could be used to determine a patient's anatomic deadspace?
   a. 1 ml/kg of ideal body weight
   b. 1 ml/lb of ideal body weight
   c. $\dot{V}_E \times \dot{V}_A$
   d. $RR \times V_T$

8. Which of the following criteria are consistent with compensated respiratory acidosis?
   a. Decreased pH; elevated PCO_2, HCO_3^- and BE
   b. Normal pH; elevated PCO_2, HCO_3^- and BE
   c. Normal pH; decreased PCO_2, HCO_3^- and BE
   d. Elevated pH, PCO_2, HCO_3^- and BE

9. Which of the following criteria are consistent with partially compensated respiratory alkalosis?
   a. Increased pH; decreased PCO_2, HCO_3^- and BE
   b. Normal pH; elevated PCO_2, HCO_3^- and BE
   c. Normal pH; decreased PCO_2, HCO_3^- and BE
   d. Increased pH; decreased PCO_2; normal HCO_3^- and BE

10. Which of the following correctly describes the chloride shift?
    a. The movement of chloride from the extracellular fluid into the intracellular fluid that occurs when the patient is acidotic from an increase in intracellular PCO_2
    b. The exchange of chloride and carbon dioxide between the red blood cell and the plasma
    c. The exchange of bicarbonate and chloride ions between the red blood cell and the plasma

11. Briefly describe the relationship between alveolar ventilation and P_aCO_2.

____

____

____

____

____

____

A patient is admitted to the pulmonary unit with increasing shortness of breath. His vital signs upon admission are BP 130/90, HR 110, RR 28, T 38.2° C. The patient is 65 years old and weighs 55 kg. The therapist performs a bedside assessment and finds that the patient has a V_T of 400 ml and $\dot{V}_E$ of 11.2 L. Use this information to answer questions 12-14.

12. What is this patient's anatomic deadspace?

____

____

____

13. a. Assuming the patient has no alveolar deadspace, what is his deadspace ventilation?

____

b. What would the patient's deadspace ventilation be if his respiratory rate decreased to 20 breaths/minute?

____

c. Explain the difference in your answers to a and b.

____

____

____

____

____

____

____

14. What is this patient's alveolar ventilation at a respiratory rate of 28?

____

15. Using the following key, identify the respiratory acid-base state for the arterial blood gases listed below:
    I. Compensated respiratory acidosis
    II. Compensated respiratory alkalosis
    III. Uncompensated respiratory acidosis
    IV. Uncompensated respiratory alkalosis
    V. Partially compensated respiratory acidosis
    VI. Partially compensated respiratory alkalosis

    a. pH 7.36, P_aCO_2 48, HCO_3^- 24, BE 0
    b. pH 7.42, P_aCO_2 29.5, HCO_3^- 18.5, BE –5.6
    c. pH 7.38, P_aCO_2 56.2, HCO_3^- 32.2, BE +4
    d. pH 7.57, P_aCO_2 21, HCO_3^- 18.7, BE –1.3
    e. pH 7.26, P_aCO_2 74, HCO_3^- 32, BE +2

Answers to Problems

1. b: Most CO_2 is transported as bicarbonate ion.
   d: CO_2 is carried as carbamino hemoglobin on reduced hemoglobin.
   f: CO_2 is carried on the hemoglobin in chemical combination with amino acids (carbamino compounds).
   g: CO_2 is carried physically dissolved in the plasma. The amount dissolved is directly related to the P_aCO_2 tension.

2. b: Arterial PCO_2 is inversely proportional to alveolar ventilation. This relationship is essential in assessing the patient's respiratory acid-base balance. If the patient is hypoventilating, then he/she shows respiratory acidosis. If the patient is hyperventilating, then he/she shows respiratory alkalosis. The degree of compensation depends upon the length of time that the acid-base condition has existed in the individual.

3. a: Mixed venous CO_2 is a reservoir for CO_2 in the blood. If $\dot{V}_A$ and alveolar perfusion does not change and mixed venous CO_2 content increases, the pressure gradient from the blood to the alveoli increases resulting in greater diffusion of CO_2 into the alveoli. This increases alveolar PCO_2.

4. b: If $\dot{V}_A$ and mixed venous CO_2 content does not change and alveolar perfusion decreases, alveolar capillary blood flow will decrease. This creates an increase in "relative" alveolar deadspace (ventilation with reduced perfusion) and alveolar PCO_2 decreases.

5. b: This is one of several formulas for calculating deadspace ventilation. For example, if the patient had no alveolar deadspace, one could take the patient's anatomic deadspace and multiply it by the respiratory frequency. The product is deadspace ventilation.

6. a: This is one of several formulas for calculating alveolar ventilation. For example, if one measured the patient's tidal volume and subtracted the anatomic deadspace, the product is alveolar ventilation for that one breath. Answer a is similar, although in place of tidal volume, minute volume and minute deadspace ventilation are used. The answer represents alveolar ventilation per minute instead of alveolar ventilation for one breath.

7. b: Another way to calculate a patient's anatomic deadspace is to find the patient's ideal body weight in kilograms and multiply that value by 2.2 ml/kg. Either technique is correct.

8. b: Compensated respiratory acidosis is a chronic hypoventilatory condition. The renal system has sufficient time to retain HCO_3^- which would result in an increased base excess. These changes normalize the pH.

9. a: Partially compensated respiratory alkalosis is a subacute hyperventilatory condition. The renal system is starting to compensate, which is manifested by a decreased bicarbonate, negative base excess and an elevated pH. The changes are not able to return the pH to normal, but compensation is occurring.

10. c: Chloride moves from the plasma into the erythrocyte when the bicarbonate that is formed in the erythrocyte diffuses into the plasma.

11. PCO_2 is inversely proportional to alveolar ventilation. When alveolar ventilation decreases, this increases the patient's alveolar PCO_2 which then increases the arterial PCO_2. Conversely, if alveolar ventilation increases, then the alveolar PCO_2 will climb. In turn, this causes the arterial PCO_2 to increase.

12. 121 ml: 55 kg $\times$ 2.2 ml/kg $=$ 121 ml

13. a. 279 ml or 7.812 L: Alveolar ventilation can be expressed either per breath (279 ml) or per minute.

    b. 2.420 L $\dot{V}_A$: The absolute amount of anatomic deadspace ventilation doesn't change, but the volume per minute is decreased when the respiratory rate decreases. The $\dot{V}_A$ decreases from 3.388 L (rate of 28) to 2.420 (rate of 20).

    c. Deadspace ventilation per minute is directly affected by changes in respiratory rate. The absolute amount of anatomic deadspace is fixed because it is determined by ideal body weight. If the patient's respiratory rate changes, it will change the minute deadspace volume because anatomic deadspace is a component of each breath. If the patient is breathing more frequently, the anatomic deadspace will also increase and ventilation will become more inefficient. When respiratory rate decreases, deadspace ventilation decreases and has less impact on alveolar ventilation.

14. 7.812 L: The patient's minute ventilation was 11.2 L; and the deadspace ventilation was 3.388 L. The difference is alveolar ventilation.

15. a. III: Uncompensated respiratory acidosis
    b. II: Compensated respiratory alkalosis
    c. I: Compensated respiratory acidosis
    d. VI: Partially compensated respiratory alkalosis
    e. V: Partially compensated respiratory acidosis

Case Study

A 70-year-old white male comes to the hospital emergency room complaining of nausea, vomiting and chest pain. His current problem began yesterday with the onset of nausea and black vomitus. The patient was admitted 4 months ago for similar complaints with a diagnosis of erosive duodenitis and some gastritis. The patient denies alcohol abuse and he is taking an H_2 blocker and a sucralfate-type drug. He denies taking any other medication.

Past Medical History:
Erosive duodenitis and gastritis
Subendocardial MI 5 months ago
COPD
Pneumonia requiring hospitalization

Social History:
Married 2 times but is single currently
+ Smoking history > 150 pack/year
– ETOH (history of abuse)

Physical Exam:
Height 5'5", Weight 120 lbs (ideal body weight 137 lbs)
Having multiple episodes of emesis of coffee ground material

Vital signs: T = normal
BP = 160/94
HR = 88
RR = 18

Respiratory: Inspiratory and expiratory rhonchi, poor cough reflex

Abdomen: Soft and tender to palpation in the midepigastrium and the right upper quadrant

CV: Sinus rhythm at 88 with a 30 degrees axis
LAD and ST-T changes suggestive of ischemia

Laboratory:
WBC: 13.1, Hb 16.8, Hct 48.4, Platelets 334,000, prothrombin time and partial thromboplastin time WNL

CXR: No infiltrates but COPD changes noted

ABGs: pH 7.47, P_aCO_2 25, P_aO_2 99, HCO_3^- 18 mMol/L, BE –5.3, S_aO_2 .98 on room air

Clinical Impression: Upper GI bleed with hematemesis; hemoconcentration with a history of duodenitis

Clinical Course: The patient continues to have hematemesis for the first 5 days of his hospitalization. He also exhibits signs of alcohol withdrawal. It is postulated that the patient is aspirating gastric contents because of his poor cough reflex. Vigorous pulmonary care is given and despite all efforts, on day 5, the patient requires intubation and mechanical ventilation (ABGs: pH 7.49, P_aCO_2 34, P_aO_2 51, S_aO_2 81%, HCO_3^- 26, BE +1.3). Weaning is attempted on day 7 with the following pulmonary function results: $\dot{V}_E$ 13.2 L, V_T 400 ml, RR 33, PIP –26 cm H_2O.

---

1. What is the respiratory acid-base classification for the patient's admitting arterial blood gases?

2. What is this patient's anatomic deadspace?

3. What is the respiratory acid-base classification for the patient's arterial blood gases before intubation?

4. Using the pulmonary function measurements during the weaning attempt, calculate the following:
   a. Deadspace ventilation (assume no alveolar deadspace)
   b. Alveolar ventilation

Answers to Case Study Questions

1. Partially compensated respiratory alkalosis: This patient has been in this acid-base state for at least 24 hours as evidenced by the lower HCO_3^- and BE.

2. 137 ml: This patient is not at his ideal weight. Deadspace must be determined by the ideal weight. If you used his actual weight you would underestimate his anatomic deadspace. The low end of the normal range for ideal body weight of a man with a medium frame is 137-148 lbs.

3. Uncompensated respiratory alkalosis: This patient's CO_2 has increased by 9 mmHg which indicates that his alveolar ventilation has decreased. This may be the result of increasing ventilatory impairment secondary to aspiration pneumonia. Even though we have not concentrated on oxygenation in this chapter, it should be mentioned that he is in oxygenation failure because of his low P_aO_2.

4. a. $\dot{V}_D$ = 4.521 L: IBW = 137 lbs, RR 33 b/min
   33 breaths/min × 137 ml/breath = $\dot{V}_A$ ml/min
   b. $\dot{V}_A$ = 8.679 L: $\dot{V}_E$ = 13.2, $\dot{V}_D$ = 4.521
   13.2 L − 4.521 L = 8.679

Suggested Additional Readings

Kacmarek, RM, Mack, CW and Dimas, S, *The Essentials of Respiratory Care,* 3rd edition, C.V. Mosby, St. Louis, MO, 1990, pp. 157-160, 170-173.

Shapiro, BA, Kacmarek, RM, Cane, RD, Peruzzi, WT and Hauptman, D, *Clinical Application of Respiratory Care,* 4th edition, Mosby-Year Book, St. Louis, MO, 1991, pp. 43-45, 233-240.

CHAPTER 4

Arterial Oxygenation

Objectives

After reading Chapter 4 and successfully completing this chapter of the workbook the student will be able to:

1. Define the following terms:

affinities	oxygen content
anaerobic metabolism	oxyhemoglobin component
Bohr effect	oxidized
clinical oxygenation assessment	oxygen dissociation curve
	partial pressure (tension)
conducting airways	partial pressure gradient
cyanosis	pathophysiology
dissolved oxygen	phosphorylase
driving force	P_IO_2
equilibration	PO_2
Haldane effect	P_{50}
heme	RBC
hemoglobin	sigmoid curve
hemolyzed	standard body temperature
globin	shift to the right
gravity-dependent	shift to the left
hemoglobinopathies	tissue hypoxia
linear	volumes percent
non-linear	2,3 DPG

2. Describe the following chemistry and physics concepts:
   a. atmospheric pressure
   b. Bunsen solubility coefficient
   c. covalent bond
   d. ferric
   e. ferrous
   f. Henry's Law
   g. imidazole
   h. peptide chains
      - alpha
      - beta
      - gamma
   i. polypeptide
   j. pyrrole ring
   k. valence
3. Describe the different effects on oxygen transport of the following types of hemoglobin:
   a. HbA
   b. HbF
   c. HbCO
   d. HbMet
4. Discuss the factors that influence oxygen affinity and their effects on the oxyhemoglobin dissociation curve.
5. Differentiate between anaerobic and aerobic metabolism.
6. Define *tissue hypoxia* in terms of ability to meet metabolic demands.
7. List the ways in which oxygen is carried in the blood.
8. Discuss the structure and importance of the hemoglobin molecule.
9. Discuss the chemical properties of the hemoglobin molecule and its constituent parts.
10. List and describe the effects of the most prevalent species of normal hemoglobin.
11. Discuss each of the normal hemoglobins and their affinities for oxygen.
12. Explain the Bohr and Haldane effects.
13. Describe the effect of oxygen and the pH of the hemoglobin.
14. Using Henry's Law, discuss gas equilibration between the alveoli and the pulmonary capillary.
15. Describe the importance of the sigmoid shape of the oxyhemoglobin dissociation curve.
16. Describe the concept of and the normal value of the P_{50} value.
17. Describe the oxygen carrying capacity of hemoglobin and compare this with the amount of dissolved oxygen in the blood.
18. Indicate both the causes and the effects of right and left shifts in the oxyhemoglobin dissociation curve.
19. Differentiate between the "ideal" lung model and the "normal" lung model.
20. Identify and explain the pathophysiologic causes of hypoxemia.
21. Explain the concept of dynamic equilibrium and alveolar oxygen tension.
22. Explain the concept of dynamic equilibrium and oxygen extraction from the alveoli.
23. Explain the effects of increased capillary perfusion on oxygen extraction from the alveoli.
24. Name and describe the three major causes of decreases in mixed venous oxygen content.
25. Discuss the $\dot{V}/\dot{Q}$ relationship and its variances.
26. Discuss the body's compensatory mechanisms for hypoxemia.

Definitions

affinity The ability to attract and hold another substance.

aerobic metabolism Cellular energy production using oxygen.

anaerobic metabolism Cellular energy production without the use of oxygen.

atmospheric pressure Pressure exerted by the atmosphere at sea level (760 mmHg, 14.7 lb/sq in).

Bohr effect A characteristic of the oxyhemoglobin dissociation curve wherein the curve shifts to the left due to the addition of CO_2 to the blood, which results in the release of more oxygen from raising the PO_2 at lower saturations.

Bunsen solubility coefficient A method of expressing the relative potential for a substance (solute) to dissolve in a fluid (solvent).

clinical oxygenation assessment Methods of assessing oxygenation which do not require access to research laboratory facilities; those evaluations which can be performed at a community hospital.

conducting airways The portions of the lungs which act as distribution pathways for inspired and expired gases but which don't take part in gas exchange.

covalent bond Chemical bonds in which two or more atoms share electrons.

cyanosis A symptom of desaturated hemoglobin which presents as a bluish coloration of the skin or mucous membranes. This is not a reliable sign either by its presence or by its absence.

dissolved oxygen Oxygen which is dissolved in the blood plasma and which exerts a partial pressure.

driving force (pressure) The pressure gradient which exists between two points in a system. Driving pressure has both magnitude and direction (vector). Driving Force (pressure) = $P_{Hi} - P_{Lo}$.

equilibration/equilibrium A state in which a balance is maintained between two systems such that when one system changes, the other system also changes to maintain the balanced state.

ferric An ionic state of the element iron (Fe) in which the positive charge equals plus 3 (Fe^{+++}).

ferrous An ionic state of the element iron (Fe) in which the positive charge equals plus 2 (Fe^{++}).

globin The base or central portion of the hemoglobin molecule to which the heme components are attached; a complex polypeptide.

gravity-dependent areas of the lung The lung zones where the distribution of both perfusion and ventilation is the greatest. The gravity-dependent areas change according to the individual's body position. In the erect position, dependent lung regions are in the bases. In the supine position, dependent areas are located in the posterior aspects of the lung.

Haldane effect A characteristic of the oxyhemoglobin dissociation curve wherein the curve shifts to the right due to the addition of O_2 to the blood, which results in the release of carbon dioxide from the hemoglobin.

HbA Adult hemoglobin; one of the normal species of hemoglobin.

HbF Fetal hemoglobin; a normal species of hemoglobin found in newborn infants.

HbCO Carboxyhemoglobin; a normal hemoglobin caused by carbon monoxide binding to heme receptor sites, which blocks O_2 binding.

HbMet Methemoglobin; a normal hemoglobin species.

heme The side chain molecules, four of which are bound to the globin component of hemoglobin and which, in turn, form a bonding site for oxygen molecules.

hemoglobin A complex polypeptide molecule whose purpose is to act as a transport mechanism for oxygen.

hemoglobinopathies Abnormal hemoglobin species with nonfunctional or dysfunctional oxygen carrying capacities.

hemolyzed Blood in which the red cell wall has ruptured, releasing hemoglobin into the plasma.

Henry's Law At a given temperature, the amount of gas that can be dissolved in a liquid is proportional to the partial pressure of the gas to which the liquid is exposed.

left shift The curve shifts to the left, towards the Y axis, indicating an increase in hemoglobin's affinity for oxygen at a given P_aO_2.

linear In a straight line.

non-linear In a curved or a random fashion.

oxygen content The total amount of oxygen, expressed in ml/dL, being carried in the blood, both combined with hemoglobin and dissolved in the plasma.

oxyhemoglobin component That part of the circulating blood volume which is composed of HbO_2.

oxidized A compound or substance which has combined with oxygen.

oxygen dissociation curve A theoretical curve plotting oxygen saturation against partial pressure of oxygen. This curve is a sigmoid (S-shaped) curve.

partial pressure (tension) The force exerted by gases dissolved in liquids. This is proportional to their proportion of the total gas concentration in the liquid.

partial pressure gradient The difference between the partial pressure of a gas in one part of a system and the partial pressure in another part of the system.

pathophysiology Changes in biologic systems caused by disease processes.

peptide chain A sequence of amino acids; a protein molecule bonded in a linear manner. **Alpha** is nomenclature for a specific bonding site on an organic molecule. Other sites include **beta** and **gamma**.

phosphorylase An enzyme which breaks phosphor bonds and releases energy for metabolic needs.

polypeptide A polypeptide chain consists of amino acids linked in a linear fashion; these are protein molecules.

porphyrin ring A complex organic molecule made up of four pyrrole rings linked by shared carbon bonds (methylene bridges).

pyrrole An organic chemical compound with four carbon atom bonds and one ammonium (NH) complex. This ring has six free bonding sites.

P_IO_2 Partial pressure of inspired oxygen.

PO_2 Partial pressure of oxygen (source unspecified).

P_{50} Partial pressure at which the blood is 50% saturated with oxygen. In normal plasma the P_{50} = 27 mmHg.

RBC Red blood cell (the cellular storage/transport unit for hemoglobin).

right shift The curve shifts to the right, away from the Y axis, indicating a decreased affinity (attraction) for oxygen by the hemoglobin at a given P_aO_2.

sigmoid curve An S-shaped curve.

standard body temperature 37° Celsius, 98.6° Fahrenheit, 310° Kelvin.

tissue hypoxia An insufficient amount of oxygen for the tissue to perform its functions without resorting to anaerobic metabolism.

valence An indicator of the binding power of a molecule or atom. The valence represents the number of unmatched electrons in the outer shell of the substance.

volumes percent The number of units of a solute in 100 ml of the solvent, e.g., the number of grams of oxygen in 100 ml of blood.

2,3 DPG 2,3 diphosphoglycerate; a biochemical.

Introduction

In this chapter Shapiro discusses the physical and chemical characteristics of the hemoglobin molecule. This is a complex subject and will require the student to commit to actively study the material in order to gain a thorough understanding of this important information.

The chapter begins with a discussion of arterial oxygenation and the determinants of tissue hypoxia. Tissue hypoxia results from inadequate tissue oxygenation and causes anaerobic metabolism within those tissues. Tissue hypoxia cannot be directly measured but must be diagnosed based on clinical judgements.

Shapiro next discusses the concept of oxygen content (CO). Oxygen content is the amount of oxygen (O_2) carried in 100 ml of blood (ml/dL). CO has two components: the oxygen dissolved in the plasma (PO_2) and the oxygen bound to hemoglobin (SO_2). Of the two, the oxygen dissolved in the plasma is a much smaller amount than the bound portion.

A detailed discussion of hemoglobin (Hb) and its chemical, physical and physiologic principles follows the discussion of hemoglobin.

Hemoglobin is the main component of the red blood cell (RBC) and is responsible for carrying the majority of the oxygen in the blood. Oxygenated hemoglobin (HbO) is what makes the blood red in color. Each RBC contains about 280 million Hb molecules, each of which carries four iron molecules, each capable of binding to an oxygen molecule.

Chemically, hemoglobin is a complex organic molecule consisting of a long, chainlike molecule called *globin* and four ring-shaped molecules called *heme*. Heme is formed by covalent bonding of four pyrrole rings to form a porphyrin molecule (see Figures 1, 2, and 3). When the porphyrin molecule forms a covalent bond with iron in its ionic ferrous form (Fe^{++}), heme is formed. Amino acids form chains (polypeptides) with nitrogen bonding sites at either end. These bonding sites are capable of covalent bonding. A combination of two alpha and two beta chains results in the formation of a globin molecule.

When four heme molecules combine with a globin molecule, the complex hemoglobin molecule is formed by covalent bonding of the polypeptide to the Fe^{++} electron. At this point five of the six free electrons in the Fe^{++} outer shell are bound, four to heme and one to globin. The sixth electron is available for reversible bonding with oxygen or other substances.

Shapiro next discusses three common Hb variants: HbF, HbCO and HbMet. *HbF*, fetal hemoglobin, is found in newborn infants and accounts for up to 85% of their hemoglobin. Unlike adult hemoglobin (HbA), HbF has two alpha and two gamma polypeptide chains. The gamma chains are thought to increase the HbF - O_2 affinity.

HbCO, carboxyhemoglobin, is formed when carbon monoxide (CO) is combined with hemoglobin. The CO forms a strong covalent bond with the Fe^{++} ion. This affinity for hemoglobin is 200-250 times the affinity that oxygen has for hemoglobin. The CO's presence on the heme blocks the oxygen from bonding. The relative attractiveness of hemoglobin for these gases is partially a product of the gas's partial pressures.

HbMet, methemoglobin, is a variant which results when the Fe^{++} ion is oxidized into the ferric (Fe^{+++}) state. In this state all of the bonding sites are taken up and oxygen can not bind to the heme. (The extra $^{+}$ indicates that three of the eight electron positions in the outer shell of the Fe atom are filled.) Additionally, the oxidation of the Fe^{++} causes the blood to take on a brownish color.

Having discussed the structure, function and common variations of the hemoglobin molecule, Shapiro next discusses the Bohr and Haldane effects. He starts by describing the acid-base changes that occur in the Hb molecule as the Hb changes its oxygenation status. As Hb is oxygenated it becomes a stronger acid than when it loses oxygen. As Hb releases O_2 at the tissue, it becomes a weaker acid, allowing it to gain hydrogen (H^+); in the lungs the binding of Hb with oxygen acidifies the Hb, reducing its affinity for H^+. This is one way that the body controls the carbamino and the bicarbonate ion mechanisms.

The *Bohr effect* refers to the addition of CO_2 to the blood in order to increase O_2 release by hemoglobin at the tissues. The *Haldane effect* refers to the addition of O_2 to the blood to effect the release of CO_2 from the hemoglobin in the lungs.

The hemoglobin dissociation curve is the next topic addressed in the text. *Henry's Law* dictates that when a liquid is exposed to a mixture of gases (atmosphere), the partial pressures of gases dissolved in liquids will equilibrate with the pressures of those gases in the atmosphere. In blood, the initial response to exposure to oxygen is for the oxygen molecules to attach to the hemoglobin. This does not directly increase PO_2. However, as the oxygen molecules cross the capillary to the RBC, some of the O_2 dissolves in the plasma, establishing the PO_2. Oxygen moves across the alveolar capillary membrane until equilibrium is reached. When the blood PO_2 is equilibrated with the alveolar (atmospheric) PO_2, the hemoglobin is fully saturated for that PO_2.

For PO_2s between 1 and 100 mmHg, the relationship between PO_2 and S_aO_2 can be describe as a sigmoid (S-shaped) curve. This curve is called the hemoglobin dissociation curve or the *oxyhemoglobin dissociation curve*. Key values for the P_aO_2 - S_aO_2 relationship are found in Table 2. It is important to note that the P_aO_2 - S_aO_2 relationship is not linear.

The normal range of hemoglobin concentration in adults is 14-16 grams per 100 ml of blood (gm/dL or gm%.) One can determine the oxygenation status of the blood if one knows the S_aO_2 or P_aO_2.

Oxygen content is further explored by Shapiro in the next section of Chapter 4. Shapiro reminds us that O_2 content is the amount of oxygen present in 100 ml of blood. He states that O_2 content is the sum of the bound plus the dissolved oxygen in a 100 ml sample of blood. Further, it is stressed that the dissolved oxygen is a small fraction of the total O_2 content. The hemoglobin is able to bind with 1.34 ml of oxygen per gram of intact hemoglobin. Calculations derived from the solubility coefficient for oxygen allow determination of the dissolved component of the O_2 content.

For each 100 ml of blood at BTPS, 0.003 ml of oxygen will dissolve per mmHg PO_2. Thus for a PO_2 of 100 mmHg, 0.3 ml of O_2 can be dissolved in 100 ml of blood (0.3 vol% or 0.3 ml/dL). While only 1-3% of the total O_2 content is dissolved in the plasma, this volume is critical as it creates the driving pressure of the P_aO_2.

Shifts of the oxyhemoglobin dissociation curve are covered next, with the following points being made: first, a shift of the curve indicates that something has altered the relationship between the S_aO_2 and the P_aO_2, signified by a change in the oxygen affinity. Second, shifts *to the right* can be caused by temperature and H^+ ion increases (decreased pH, increased PCO_2). Shifts *to the left*, on the other hand, are caused by increased pH, decreased PCO_2 (decreased H^+ ion concentration) and decreased temperature.

Shifts to the right signal decreased oxygen - hemoglobin affinity. This should promote improved tissue oxygenation since the hemoglobin will give up oxygen more readily. However, large shifts to the right may reduce the ability of hemoglobin to carry sufficient oxygen, reducing O_2 content. Shifts to the left indicate that the hemoglobin has an increased affinity for oxygen. This means that the hemoglobin is less likely to give oxygen to the tissues since it could be considered to be more tightly bound to the hemoglobin.

The concept of P_{50} is discussed next. Shapiro defines P_{50} as the oxygen tension at which the hemoglobin is 50% saturated at 37° C, the P_aCO_2 is 40 mmHg, and the pH is 7.40. The clinical value of the P_{50} is questionable. The factors which commonly affect oxygen - hemoglobin affinity don't change P_{50}. Normal P_{50} is 27 mmHg. Lower values of P_{50} indicate increased affinity, such as that caused by decreased 2,3 DPG levels, resulting in a "tighter" oxyhemoglobin bond inhibiting release of O_2 at the tissues. Stored blood often has decreased 2,3 DPG levels.

The ideal lung model as described by Shapiro would have no deadspace ventilation (all alveoli would be ventilated), and all blood from the right ventricle would pass through perfect pulmonary capillaries where diffusion across the alveolar capillary membrane would be unimpeded. Given these conditions, the ideal inspired oxygen tension (P_IO_2) would be:

$$(P_B \times F_IO_2) = (760 \times 0.209) = 160 \text{ mmHg}$$

The ideal alveolar oxygen tension P_AO_2 would be:

$$(P_B \times PH_2O) \times F_IO_2 - (P_ACO_2/RQ) =$$
$$(760 - 47) \times 0.209 - (40 \text{ mmHg}/0.8) =$$
$$(713 \times 0.209) - 50 =$$
$$100 \text{ mmHg}$$

Ideal arterial oxygen tension (P_aO_2) would equal the ideal alveolar tension since equilibrium would be reached so that $P_aO_2 = P_AO_2$.

The situation in the normal lung model is not as neat and clear, since both shunt and deadspace ventilation exist due to uneven distribution of ventilation and perfusion and the presence of deadspace ventilation and anatomic shunts. As a result of these factors, the blood entering the left ventricle is not as well-oxygenated as possible. Although this A-a oxygen gradient is unimportant in normal individuals, pathologic variations of these ventilation and perfusion factors can lead to significant oxygenation deficits.

A discussion of the pathophysiologic causes of hypoxemia reveals that several key factors, operating either singly or in combination, can cause hypoxemia (a relative deficiency of oxygen in the blood). The point is made that cyanosis is not a reliable index of hypoxemia in all patients. Cyanosis is usually associated with greater than 5 gm/dL of reduced (unoxygenated) hemoglobin, and its detection may be dependent on visual perception and ambient lighting conditions. Anemic patients may be very desaturated without cyanosis, while patients with polycythemia may be cyanotic with normal O_2 tensions.

Alterations of arterial oxygenation must be caused by one or more of the following:

- reduced P_AO_2
  - decreased V_{alv}
  - decreased F_IO_2
- reduced alveolar oxygen extraction
  - decreased capillary blood flow
  - increased $C\bar{v}O_2$

Pulmonary artery oxygen saturation (mixed venous SO_2) is best reflected by oxyhemoglobin saturation. Changes in $S\bar{v}O_2$ reflect the O_2 needed to maintain A-a O_2 equilibrium. The relationship between $S\bar{v}O_2$ and O_2 needs is inverse; as $S\bar{v}O_2$ decreases, O_2 needs decrease.

Hemoglobin concentration reflects a direct relationship with O_2 needed to maintain equilibrium; as [Hb] increases, more O_2 is need to effect A-a equilibrium. Similarly, increasing capillary perfusion per unit of time will increase the need for available oxygen as more unsaturated Hb will be exposed to the alveoli per unit of time.

Decreased $S\bar{v}O_2$ has three major causes: increased metabolism, decreased cardiac output and decreased S_aO_2. The best way to reverse this process is to increase cardiac output.

Pulmonary shunt is blood that does not take part in oxygenation. There are two major types of pulmonary shunts: anatomic and capillary. Anatomic shunt is blood that goes from right to left heart without passing through the pulmonary capillaries. Capillary shunts are blood flows that are directed through pulmonary capillaries which pass unventilated alveoli. Both of these situations are referred to as *zero* $\dot{V}/\dot{Q}$ since no exposure to the oxygen in alveolar gas takes place. The hypoxic effect of any shunt depends on the size of the shunt and the oxygenation status of the shunted blood.

Deficits in oxygen diffusion represent another cause of hypoxemia. These deficits can be caused by scarring or increases in the alveolar capillary membrane width. Diffusion deficits are responsive to increased alveolar F_IO_2.

Compensation for hypoxemia is dependent on the proper function of the peripheral PO_2 chemoreceptors in the carotid and aortic bodies. These receptors sense tissue PO_2 level changes and signal the brain through their afferent (sensory) nerves. The brain then signals the heart and lungs through efferent nerve (motor) channels to increase ventilation and cardiac output.

Key Points

- Tissue hypoxia exists when cellular oxygen supply fails to meet metabolic needs.
- Assessment of tissue hypoxia is a clinical judgement.
- Tissue hypoxia requires that the cell use anaerobic metabolism.
- Oxygen is carried in the blood either in solution (dissolved) in the plasma or bound to hemoglobin (oxyhemoglobin).
- The volume of oxygen in 100 ml of blood is called the oxygen content; this includes both dissolved and bound oxygen.
- Most oxygen carried in the blood is bound to hemoglobin.
- Only about 1-3% of the oxygen in the blood is carried in solution.
- The oxyhemoglobin component is measured as a ratio of the amount of hemoglobin actually carried to the amount that the hemoglobin could carry. This ratio is called the oxygen saturation (O_2 sat or SO_2).
- Hemoglobin which is not fully component with O_2 is called reduced hemoglobin (Hbr).
- The dissolved component is measured as the partial pressure of oxygen (PO_2).
- In humans, hemoglobin is the main component of the red blood cell (RBC) and when oxygenated causes the red color of blood.
- Each RBC can carry 280 million hemoglobin molecules.

Facts About Hemoglobin

- Each hemoglobin molecule has four iron atoms.
- Hemoglobin is a very large and complex molecule whose exact structure is not known.
- Hemoglobin consists of two types of molecules: heme, a relatively small molecule, and globin, a long, large chain of protein (polypeptide).
- Four heme molecules bond to one globin molecule to make the complex hemoglobin molecule.
- The heme molecule consists of four covalently bonded pyrrole rings whose nitrogen atoms share bonds with an iron (ferrous) ion.

- After bonding to form the heme molecule, the Fe^{++} (ferrous) ion has used four of its six valence bonding sites, leaving two sites available for covalent bonding.
- One of the remaining bonding sites on the Fe^{++} ion forms a bond with the globin molecule, and the sixth is available for bonding with oxygen.
- The sixth covalent heme bond is a reversible bond with oxygen.
- Abnormal amino acid sequences in the polypeptide (protein) chains may result in abnormal types of hemoglobin (hemoglobinopathies), causing disturbances of the oxygen carrying mechanism.

Hemoglobin Variants

- The relatively frequent variants of hemoglobin are fetal (HbF), carboxy (HbCO) and methemoglobin (HbMet).
- About 85% of the hemoglobin found in neonates has globin molecules comprised of two alpha and two gamma protein chains rather than the alpha and beta chains found in HbA.
- The presence of the gamma chains in HbF appears to increase O_2 affinity and may reduce the activity of phosphorylase enzyme systems in the RBC.
- HbCO is created when carbon monoxide (CO) forms covalent bonds with the ferrous ion.
- CO has 200-500 times more affinity for hemoglobin than does oxygen.
- When CO is bonded to heme, there is no room for O_2 to bond.
- The partial pressure of the gases to which the hemoglobin is exposed affects the affinity of hemoglobin for those gases.
- The greater the partial pressure of O_2, the lower the affinity of hemoglobin for CO, and vice versa.
- Oxidation of the Fe^{++} (ferrous) ion to the Fe^{+++} (ferric) ionic state results in the production of HbMet.
- An easy way to remember the cause of HbMet production is to recall that HbMet is brownish (rusty) in color. Rust is a form of oxidation, which is what happens to the Fe^{++} ion.
- HbMet decreases the bonding sites available for O_2 attachment.

Acid-base Effects on Hemoglobin

- Oxygenated hemoglobin is a stronger acid than deoxygenated hemoglobin.
- Release of oxygen to the tissues changes the acid-base status of the hemoglobin to a weaker acid, allowing the hemoglobin to combine with H^+ ions.
- As O_2 is picked up in the pulmonary circulation, the Hb becomes more acidic and less capable of combining with H^+.
- The changes in hemoglobin acid-base status aid in the reversal of the bicarbonate and carbamino mechanisms, enhancing CO_2 elimination.
- The *Bohr effect* is the addition of CO_2 to the blood to increase O_2 release from the hemoglobin.
- The *Haldane effect* refers to the addition of O_2 to the blood to increase the release of CO_2 from the hemoglobin.
- These effects are another way of describing the biochemical relationships among hemoglobin, oxygen and carbon dioxide.

The Hemoglobin Dissociation Curve

- The dissociation of oxygen from hemoglobin is determined by application of Henry's Law.
- Henry's Law states that the partial pressures of gases in a solution will be equal to the partial pressures in the gas to which the gas is exposed.
- Plotting the P_aO_2 of plasma against the % saturation of plasma results in a sigmoid (S-shaped) curve at physiologic temperatures and pressures for PO_2 values between 1 and 100 mmHG.
- At normal temperatures the plasma is 50% saturated at 27 mmHg P_aO_2. (See Table 2 for additional critical points on the O_2 dissociation curve.)
- The range of normal values for Hb in adults is 12-16 grams per 100 ml of blood (12-16 gm/dL or gm%).

Oxygen Content

- Oxygen content is defined as the amount of O_2 in 100 ml of blood. This consists of both the bound and the dissolved oxygen.
- The majority of the O_2 in blood is bound to hemoglobin. Only a fraction of the O_2 (1-3%) is dissolved in the plasma.
- 1 gram of HbA is capable of carrying 1.34 ml of O_2 when 100% saturated.
- The amount of O_2 dissolved in plasma is dependent on its solubility coefficient.
- At BTPS, 0.003 ml of O_2 can be dissolved in 100 ml of blood per mmHg PO_2.

- For a PO_2 of 100 mmHg, 100 ml of blood will dissolve 0.3 ml of O_2.
- Dissolved oxygen is expressed in milliliters per decaliter (ml/dL) or volumes percent (vol%).
- Increased temperature or $[H^+]$ (↑ PCO_2 and ↓ pH) shift the O_2 dissociation curve to the right, decreasing the affinity of hemoglobin for oxygen.
- Decreased temperature or $[H^+]$ (↑ pH and ↓ PCO_2) shift the O_2 dissociation curve to the left, increasing the affinity of hemoglobin for oxygen.
- Decreasing the affinity of hemoglobin for oxygen improves tissue oxygenation.
- Increasing the affinity of hemoglobin for oxygen reduces tissue oxygenation.
- P_{50} is the PO_2 at which hemoglobin is 50% saturated at pH 7.40, PCO_2 40 mmHg and temperature 37°C.
- P_{50} normally is 27 mmHg in adults.
- Decreased P_{50} indicates increased O_2 - Hb affinity.
- Decreased 2,3 DPG reduced tissue oxygenation by increasing O_2 - Hb affinity.
- P_{50} is a controversial measurement whose clinical utility may be doubtful.
- Exchange of O_2 and CO_2 is dependent on the existence of a partial pressure gradient between the gas and the blood.
- "Normal" lungs differ from "ideal" lungs in four important ways:
  - existence of deadspace ventilation (conducting airways)
  - uneven distribution of ventilation (gravity dependence)
  - uneven distribution of perfusion (gravity dependence)
  - anatomic vascular shunt (pleural, thebesian and bronchial veins)
- Although normal A-a gradient has little effect on normal subjects, the factors creating the difference can cause significant effects in the cardiopulmonary compromised patient.
- Hypoxemia is defined as a "relative deficiency of oxygen in the blood."
- Cyanosis is a bluish color of the skin, mucous membranes and nail beds caused by increased amounts of reduced hemoglobin.
- Although cyanosis has been correlated to the presence of 5 gm/dL or more of reduced hemoglobin, detection of hypoxemia by this method is unreliable due to lighting and color perception differences.
- Absence of hemoglobin does not mean that there is no tissue hypoxia.
- Patients with polycythemia (increase hemoglobin concentration) can be cyanotic while oxygenating tissues adequately.
- A low P_aO_2 must be due to either ↓ P_AO_2 or shunting ($\dot{V}/\dot{Q} = 0$) in the ideal lung.
- P_AO_2 results from the dynamic equilibrium between O_2 delivery to the alveolus and O_2 extraction from the alveolus, that is, between the tidal volume (and F_IO_2) and the venous O_2 content ($C_{\bar{v}}O_2$).
- With $C_{\bar{v}}O_2$ constant, ↓ V_{alv} and/or ↓ F_IO_2 will result in ↓ O_2 delivery to the alveoli. Increases in V_{alv} and/or F_IO_2 will ↑ alveolar O_2 delivery.
- On the other hand, if alveolar O_2 delivery factors are constant, ↓ pulmonary artery O_2 content or ↑ pulmonary capillary blood flow will increase O_2 extraction from the alveolus.
- Mixed venous O_2 content is best reflected by mixed venous O_2 saturation ($S_{\bar{v}}O_2$). ↓ $S_{\bar{v}}O_2$ increases demand for O_2 molecules in order to reach equilibrium with the P_AO_2. This is done by increasing alveolar extraction.
- As perfusion increases, so does alveolar oxygen extraction because more blood can be exposed to the alveolar oxygen reservoir in the same period of time.
- Decreased mixed venous oxygen saturation may have three prime causes: ↑ metabolic rate, ↓ cardiac output or ↓ P_aO_2. These may occur singly or in conjunction with one another.
- Low $\dot{V}/\dot{Q}$ means that perfusion exceeds ventilation (↑ $\dot{Q}$ or ↓ $\dot{V}$). This condition can lead to ↓ P_AO_2 and hypoxemia.
- Anatomic shunting refers to perfusion that does not utilize the pulmonary capillaries on its way from the right to the left heart.
- Capillary shunting is blood that goes through the pulmonary capillaries, which are near unventilated alveoli.
- The effect of both anatomic and capillary shunting is to add unoxygenated (right heart) blood into the left heart. This is also called true shunt or zero $\dot{V}/\dot{Q}$ since there is no opportunity to oxygenate the blood.
- *Shunt* and *hypoxemia* are not synonymous terms. Their relationship does not appear to be either direct or linear.
- The hypoxemic effect of a shunt is dependent on shunt size (volume) and oxygenation status of the blood.
- As perfusion time (transit time) increases, blood oxygenation worsens.

- Hypoxemic response is dependent on the body's ability to recognize the condition and improve cardiovascular and pulmonary function in order to enhance alveolar oxygenation.
- The body's ability to recognize that hypoxemia is present is dependent on the function of the peripheral carotid and aortic PO_2 chemoreceptor (bodies), which sense decreases in tissue PO_2.
- Upon sensing reduced PO_2, the carotid bodies send afferent signals to the brain. The brain then sends efferent signals to the cardiac and pulmonary systems to increase ventilation and cardiac output.
- Increasing V_{alv} is an inefficient way of ↑ P_AO_2 due to the increased work of breathing; however, increasing F_IO_2 and assisting ventilation are effective measures in reducing hypoxemia.
- The most important compensatory measure for hypoxemia is to increase cardiac output.

Formulas

Henry's Law

For any liquid, sol $\simeq$ PP(X),

where: X = a gas
PP = partial pressure
sol = solubility

Oxygen Content

$$O_2 \text{ content} = \frac{\text{dissolved } O_2 \text{ / + } O_2 \text{ bound to Hb}}{100 \text{ ml of blood}}$$

Oxygen saturation (O_2 sat or SO_2)

SO_2 = (actual HbO/potential HbO) × 100
If actual HbO = 1.25 gm O_2/gm Hb and potential HbO = 1.34 gm O_2/gm Hb,
SO_2 = (1.25/1.34) × 100 = 93.28%

Ideal Inspired PO_2 Equation

$P_B \times F_IO_2$
Example: at sea level P_B = 760 mmHg, F_IO_2 = 0.209
Ideal Inspired PO_2 = 760 × 0.209 = 159 $\simeq$ 160 mmHg

Ideal Alveolar PO_2 at BPTS

$$P_AO_2 = [(P_B - P_{H2O}) \times F_IO_2] - [(P_ACO_2/RQ)]$$
$$P_AO_2 = [(760 - 47) \times 0.21] - [(40/0.8)]$$
$$P_AO_2 = (713 \times 0.21) - 50$$
$$P_AO_2 = 149.73 - 50$$
$$P_AO_2 \simeq 100 \text{ mmHg}$$

Tables and Figures

Symbol	*Name*
HbO	Oxyhemoglobin
HbA	Adult hemoglobin
HbF	Fetal hemoglobin
HbCO	Carboxyhemoglobin
HbMet	Methemoglobin

Table 1: Common hemoglobin species.

mmHg	*% Saturation*
27	50
40	75
60	90
85	95
97	99

(PCO_2 = 40 mmHg, Temp = 37°, pH = 7.40)

Table 2: Normal oxygen saturation of Hb at various P_aO_2 levels.

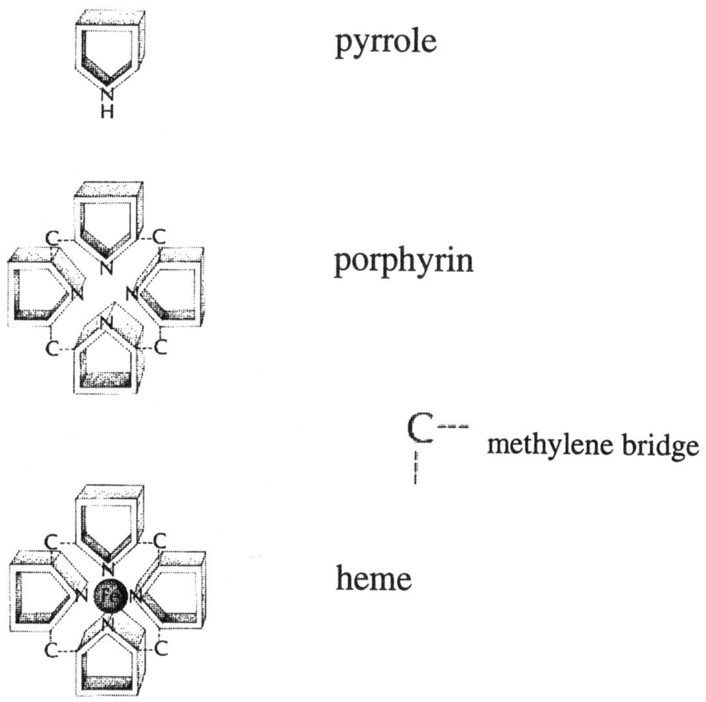

Figure 1: The chemical structure of heme.

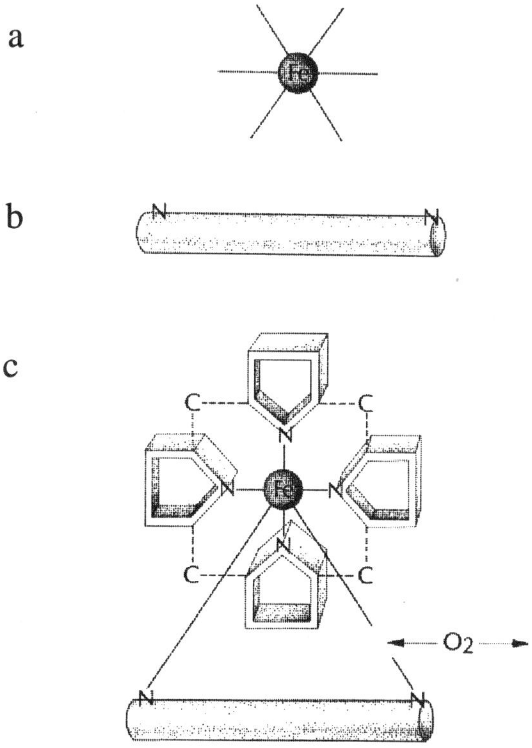

Figure 2: a, the ferrous ion (Fe^{++}) with six potential valence bonds; **b**, schematic representation of a polypeptide chain with two imidazole nitrogens that are capable of forming covalent bonds with metal ions. A protein molecule containing two alpha and two beta polypeptide chains is known as a globin molecule; **c**, heme molecule attached to polypeptide chain. Four heme molecules attached to the four polypeptide chains of a globin molecule constitute the molecule hemoglobin.

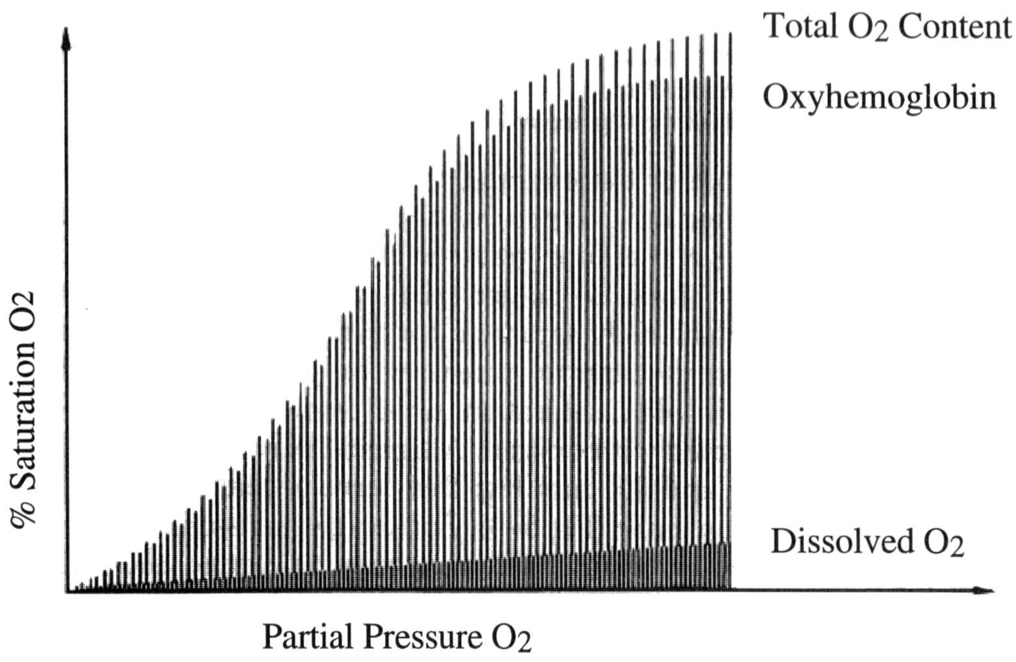

Figure 3: Oxygen content and hemoglobin saturation. Total oxygen content is shown, along with the portion attached to hemoglobin and the portion dissolved in plasma. As long as the hemoglobin is not fully saturated, great increases in oxygen content are seen with small increases in PO_2. In this range, almost all the increase in oxygen content is due to oxygen attached to hemoglobin. When hemoglobin is maximally saturated, large increases in PO_2 are accompanied by small increases in oxygen content, because only increases in dissolved oxygen are possible.

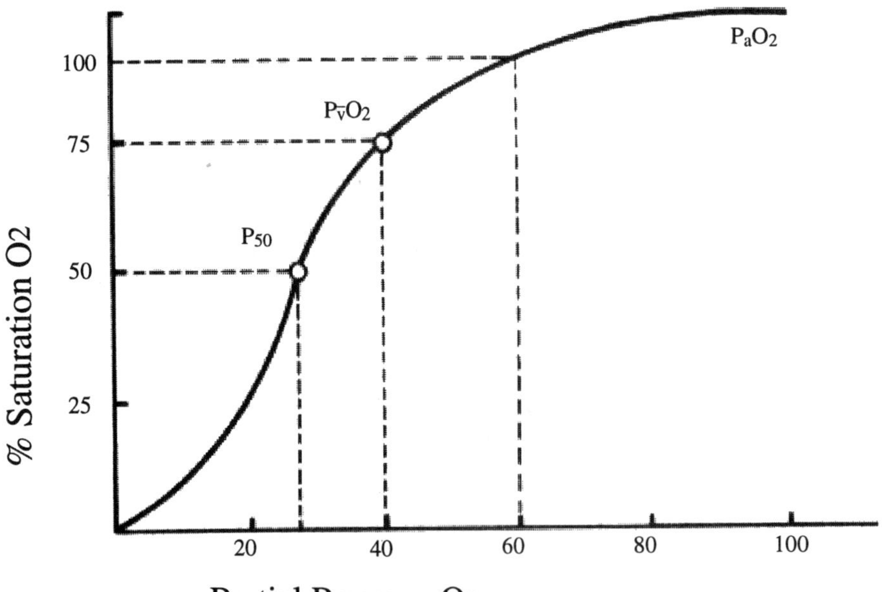

Figure 4: The hemoglobin dissociation curve. This curve shows the relationship of plasma oxygen partial pressure to the degree to which potential oxygen carrying hemoglobin sites have oxygen attached (% saturation oxygen). This nonlinear relationship accounts for most of the oxygen reserves in blood. Normally, hemoglobin is 50% saturated at a plasma PO_2 of approximately 27 mmHg; this is designated P_{50}. Normal mixed venous blood has an oxygen partial pressure ($P_{\bar{v}}O_2$) of 40 mmHg and an oxyhemoglobin saturation of 75%. A PO_2 of 60 mmHg normally results in approximately 90% saturation. Normal arterial blood has an oxygen partial pressure (P_aO_2) of 97 mmHg and an oxyhemoglobin saturation of 97%.

Problems

Select and mark the best answer.

1. Each normal hemoglobin molecule consists of a single globin component and _____ heme component(s).
   a. a single
   b. four
   c. six
   d. eight
   e. ten

2. The Haldane effect relates to the
   a. reduction in O_2 release as the plasma CO_2 increases.
   b. increase in O_2 release as the plasma CO_2 increases.
   c. reduction in CO_2 release as the plasma O_2 increases.
   d. increase in CO_2 release as the plasma O_2 increases.
   e. decrease in plasma CO_2 as bound $HbCO_2$ decreases.

3. A porphyrin ring contains four pyrrole molecules connected by methylene bonds and
   a. six di-hydrogen molecules.
   b. two ammonia complexes.
   c. four nitrogen bonding sites.
   d. one methylene tori-oxide unit.
   e. a bivalent monocholyne bond.

4. Which of the following hemoglobin types is not found in adults?
   a. Hb
   b. HbMet
   c. HbCO
   d. HbA
   e. HbF

5. Which of the following statements is true?
   a. The more oxygen on the hemoglobin, the more efficient the respiratory process.
   b. Oxygen bound to hemoglobin cannot directly change P_aO_2.
   c. Carbon dioxide cannot bind to reduced hemoglobin.
   d. Fetal hemoglobin refers to immature red cells in the bone marrow.
   e. The heme components form long chains of complex proteins.

6. The P_aO_2 is critical because it
   a. represents the majority of oxygen stores within the body.
   b. determines the driving pressure for gas exchange across the biological membranes.
   c. determines the amount of hemoglobin produced for oxygen transport to the tissues.
   d. provides the force needed to push CO_2 from the gaseous phase on to the heme molecule.
   e. is the best indicator of cellular energy levels and production.

7. At standard atmospheric pressure (P_AO_2 100 mmHg), fully saturated with water vapor (PH_2O 47 mmHg) and body temperature (37° C), what is the maximum amount of O_2 that can be dissolved in 100 ml of blood?
   a. 14.7 gm
   b. 0.003 mg
   c. 760 ml
   d. 6.03 gm
   e. 0.3 ml

8. Hemoglobin is _____ times more likely to attract carbon monoxide (CO) than oxygen.
   a. 200-250
   b. 175-225
   c. 150-200
   d. 125-175
   e. 100-150

9. O_2 content refers to the amount of oxygen carried in the blood. Which of the following best expands this definition?
   a. The majority of the oxygen content exists in the dissolved state.
   b. Only free oxygen can be classified as part of the oxygen content.
   c. All oxygen stores in the body must be calculated to determine oxygen content.
   d. Oxygen content has three components: bound to hemoglobin, dissolved and chemically combined.
   e. Oxygen content consists of the dissolved oxygen in the plasma and that bound to hemoglobin.

10. Methemoglobin is caused by
    a. the methylene bonds on the heme molecule.
    b. decreased or poor quality intake of supplemental vitamins.
    c. oxidation of the Fe^{++} atom in the heme to the Fe^{+++} state.
    d. inadequate metabolism of fetal hemoglobin by the liver.
    e. the normal aging process of the globin molecule.

11. What is the traditional oxygen carrying capacity of 1 gram of hemoglobin?
    a. 1.34 ml/gm Hb
    b. 1.39 ml/gm Hb
    c. 6.23 gm
    d. 3.1415 nanamoles
    e. 15 gm%

12. Which of the following statements best describes the Bohr effect?
    a. Methemoglobin level changes with plasma pH.
    b. Hemoglobin concentration increases as P_aCO_2 falls.
    c. As pH becomes more alkalotic, P_aO_2 increases.
    d. HCO_3^- should be twice the $(P_a - P_e)$ CO_2 difference.
    e. Increased CO_2 levels in the blood enhance O_2 release.

13. Decreased 2,3 DPG will cause which of the following conditions?
    a. A shift of the oxyhemoglobin curve to the left with reduced oxygen release to the tissues

b. A shift of the oxyhemoglobin curve to the right with reduced oxygen release to the tissues
c. A shift of the oxyhemoglobin curve to the right with increased oxygen release to the tissues
d. A shift of the oxyhemoglobin curve to the left with increased oxygen release to the tissues
e. Increased hemolysis due to the breakdown of protein chains in the globin molecule

14. P_{50} is the
a. O_2 saturation when the partial pressure of oxygen equals 50 mmHg.
b. partial pressure of oxygen where the blood is 50% saturated.
c. point at which the P_aCO_2 is half of the P_aO_2 at a given hemoglobin concentration.
d. time when half of the O_2 content is bound to hemoglobin and half dissolved in plasma.
e. oxygen consumption value when half of the metabolic oxygen stores have been used up.

15. The Haldane effect refers to
a. the enhanced release of CO_2 when the blood is well oxygenated.
b. hemoglobin retaining CO_2 in an oxygen-rich environment.
c. the conversion of Fe^{++} heme to Fe^{+++} heme in the presence of high CO_2 partial pressure.
d. the degradation of hemoglobin by oxidation in the mitochondria of the red cell.
e. the reversible color change hemoglobin undergoes when oxygenated or deoxygenated.

Answers to Problems

1. b: A normal hemoglobin molecule consists of a single globin component and four heme components which form the oxygen bonding sites.

2. c: The Haldane effect refers to the increase in CO_2 release from the hemoglobin which accompanies increased plasma O_2. This increases the partial pressure of CO_2 in the plasma, allowing for enhanced CO_2 removal through the alveolar capillary membrane.

3. c: The porphyrin is made of four pyrrole rings connected by methylene bonds and contains four nitrogen bonding sites. In this configuration a heme molecule can be constructed by addition of an Fe^{++} molecule in a covalent bond.

4. e: Hb is "reduced" (desaturated) hemoglobin, HbMet is methemoglobin where Fe^{++} has oxidized to an Fe^{+++} state, HbCO is carboxyhemoglobin (Hb combined with carbon monoxide), and HbA is adult hemoglobin. HbF is fetal hemoglobin found in newborns.

5. b: A substance must be in the gas phase in order to exert a partial pressure. When oxygen is attached to the hemoglobin, it is not in the gaseous state and thus can't exert a partial pressure. Only the dissolved oxygen is capable of being measured as a "blood gas."

6. d: PO_2 represents the pressure gradient which provides the force needed to move oxygen across the biological membranes in the tissues, cells and lungs. This pressure is produced by a small amount (1-3%) of the oxygen content. The rest of the oxygen is bound to hemoglobin and does not exert a partial pressure.

7. e: 0.003 ml of oxygen per 1 mmHg O_2 pressure per 100 ml of blood.

8. a: Carbon monoxide has 200-250 times the affinity for hemoglobin than oxygen.

9. e: Oxygen content equals the amount of oxygen dissolved in 100 ml of blood plus the amount of oxygen bound to the hemoglobin in that 100 ml of blood. The majority of oxygen in the blood is carried bound to the hemoglobin; only a small amount is dissolved in the blood plasma.

10. c: Methemoglobin is a result of the oxidation of the Fe^{++} (ferrous) ions into a Fe^{+++} (ferric) ionic state. The result is that there are no free bonding sites on the heme molecule for oxygen bonding. The exclusion of the O_2 from the hemoglobin molecule results in a brownish coloration of the blood.

11. a: The traditional oxygen carrying capacity is 1.34 milliliters of oxygen per gram of hemoglobin in intact RBCs. More recent studies have used hemolyzed RBC and have shown carrying capacities of up to 1.39 ml/gm Hb. Since the normal Hb is not hemolyzed in the blood, the classical value is more appropriate for clinical use.

12. d: The Bohr effect relates to the propensity of hemoglobin to release oxygen molecules more readily in the presence of elevated CO_2 levels in the blood. The increased CO_2 results in a more acidic environment, weakening the reversible ($Fe^{++} - O_2$) bonds in the heme complex.

13. a: Decreased 2,3 DPG shifts the oxyhemoglobin curve to the left, reducing O_2 release by the hemoglobin to the tissues and thus reducing cellular oxygen supplies. Reduced O_2 supply to the cells results in increased anaerobic metabolism, increased lactic acid production and decreased energy production.

14. b: The P_{50} is that partial pressure on the oxyhemoglobin curve where the hemoglobin in the blood is 50% saturated. In normal individuals that is at a P_aO_2 of 27 mmHg.

15. a: The Haldane effect says that addition of O_2 to the blood will increase the release of CO_2 by hemoglobin. Therefore, well-oxygenated blood will exchange CO_2 more efficiently than will poorly oxygenated blood.

Application Exercises

Each of the following patients presents a problem regarding C_aO_2, hypoxemia and/or cyanosis. Your task is to describe the problem and suggest solutions which will remediate the patient's problem.

Situation 1

Pedro Salizar is a resident of Peru who lives in the upper reaches of the Andes Mountains. Pedro is visiting the U.S. as part of a cultural exchange. Because Pedro lives "at altitude," he is normally polycythemic with a [Hb] of 20-22 mg/dL. Sr. Salizar is seen in the ER due to intestinal distress. The medical resident notes the presence of nail bed and mucosal cyanosis. The resident asks for ABGs and requests supplemental oxygenation.

1. How do you respond and why?
2. Why is his Hb status as reported above?
3. If Pedro's ABGs come back with "normal" values, how do you explain his cyanosis?
4. Is supplemental O_2 warranted? Why or why not?

Situation 2

Mrs. Yvonne Carson, 87 years old, is seen in the outpatient clinic for a complaint of generalized weakness, loss of appetite and weight loss. Mrs. Carson's husband expired two months ago, and she is reported by her children to have been "depressed." She is frail and thin with reduced skin turgor. The physician orders IV fluids and a CBC. The CBC reveals markedly decreased hemoglobin and an increased hematocrit. ABGs reveal hypoxemia, although she has no cyanosis.

1. What short-range steps should be taken to treat Mrs. Carson's hypoxemia? Explain your rationale for these steps.
2. What long-range plans need to be made to ensure a resolution of Mrs. Carson's condition?
3. Will oxygen administration alone reverse the hypoxemia Mrs. Carson is experiencing? Why or why not?

Suggested Additional Readings

Marino, PL, *The ICU Book*, Lea & Febiger, Philadelphia, PA, 1991, pp. 319-321.

Pierson, DJ and Kacmarek, RM, *Foundations of Respiratory Care*, Churchill Livingstone, New York, NY, 1992, pp. 106-113.

Wilkins, RL and Dexter, JR, *Respiratory Disease: Principles of Patient Care,* F.A. Davis, Philadelphia, PA, 1993, pp. 2-5.

CHAPTER 5

Normal Ranges and Interpretation Guidelines

Objectives

After reading Chapter 5 and successfully completing this chapter of the workbook the student will be able to:

1. Demonstrate understanding of the meaning of a bell-shaped curve when plotting data.
2. State the normal values and ranges for arterial blood gas and acid-base variables.
3. Define and explain the term *supportive therapy.*
4. Define *clinical judgement* in terms of *acceptable range.*
5. State the prediction formulas for predicting pH from acute P_aCO_2 changes.
6. Given appropriate data, solve the acute pH change formulas.
7. Explain the inverse relationship between pH and P_aCO_2.
8. Given appropriate data, calculate predicted plasma bicarbonate (HCO_3^-).
9. Explain the relationship of total ventilation to alveolar ventilation.
10. Differentiate between anatomical deadspace (V_{Danat}) and physiological deadspace (V_{Dphys}).
11. Given any two of the values for minute ventilation (MV), alveolar ventilation ($\dot{V}_A$) and deadspace ventilation ($\dot{V}_D$), calculate the third value.
12. State the effect of exercise on normal MV as it relates to metabolic rate and cardiac output.
13. Define the following terms:
    acceptable range
    arithmetic mean
    base excess/deficit
    cardiac output
    cardiopulmonary reserve
    clinical judgement
    clinical significance
    deadspace ventilation
    hypoxemia
    instrument variability
    mean
    median
    mode
    myocardial ischemia
    normal range
    prognostic
    standard deviation
    symmetrical distribution
    tachy
    95% confidence level
14. Explain the effect of exercise on $\dot{V}_A$ and P_aCO_2 in the normal individual.
15. Discuss the reasons that larger than normal MVs are required to maintain normal P_aCO_2 in ventilated patients.
16. Define the term *cardiopulmonary reserve.*
17. Explain what is meant by the phrase "minute ventilation to P_aCO_2 disparity."
18. Discuss the A-a oxygen gradient and its significance.
19. Perform calculations to compensate P_aO_2 for age.
20. State the normal values for P_aO_2, ideal P_aO_2 and F_IO_2 for an individual breathing room air at sea level.
21. Given the appropriate information, determine a patient's predicted P_aO_2.
22. With the correct data available, calculate a patient's A-a oxygen gradient at various levels of F_IO_2.
23. State the normal ranges for oxygen saturation which reflect both adequate and normal oxygenation.
24. Given initial P_aO_2 and % change in % F_IO_2, calculate the predicted P_aO_2.
25. Explain the concepts of base excess and base deficit.
26. Given the proper data, calculate the predicted respiratory component of pH.
27. Given the proper data, calculate the predicted metabolic component of pH.
28. List the guidelines for bicarbonate administration.
29. Given correct clinical data, calculate base deficit and the initial correcting dose of bicarbonate for the patient.

Definitions

acceptable range A loose, non-objective term describing a set of values which although possibly not within the "normal" range are still recognized as being reasonably appropriate and safe for the patient (see clinical judgement).

arithmetic average The average (see mean).

base excess/deficit The positive or negative deviation of the base buffer system (HCO_3^-) from the normal value at a given pH and P_aCO_2.

cardiac output ($\dot{Q}_T$) Volume of blood ejected by the heart per minute; it is a product of stroke volume multiplied by heart rate per minute.

cardiopulmonary reserve The actual ability of the cardiopulmonary system to maintain adequate function in the face of additional physiologic stress on the organism.

clinical judgement A combination of objective observation and measurement, influenced by experience and subjective impressions, which leads to a provisional diagnosis and treatment plan.

clinical significance The "real" importance of the data in terms of usefulness in a patient care situation.

deadspace ventilation The volume of inspired air which does not take part in gas exchange.

hypoxemia P_aO_2 below 80 mmHg.

instrument variability Built-in errors in measurement equipment due to sensitivity, operator perception, accuracy, variation in sampling techniques, etc.

mean The sum of the values of the data divided by the number of pieces of data (X/N where X = sum of the values and N = number of data items).

median The middle value in a set of ranked data.

myocardial ischemia Decreased or absent oxygenated blood flow to the heart muscle.

normal range Values for mean and standard deviations of lab tests gathered from very large groups of subjects. Usually expressed as +/– 2 SD from the mean value (23 +/– 6).

prognostic Predicted outcome or able to predict outcome, or as the range of the SDs (17-29).

standard deviation A measure of the spread or distribution of a set of data around the mean. 1 standard deviation (1 SD) represents the distribution of $\simeq$ 65% of the data, 2 SD represents the spread of $\simeq$ 95%, 3 SD $\simeq$ 99%.

symmetrical distribution Infers equal spread on either side of the midpoint; mirror image; e.g., the human body has symmetrical distribution when right and left halves are compared.

tachy A prefix meaning "fast" or "rapid"; e.g., tachycardia means "rapid heart rate."

95% confidence level Equivalent to the 2nd SD; that is, there is a 95% chance that the data did not occur by chance alone.

Introduction

Chapter 5 begins with a discussion of the need for objective data when evaluating and treating patients. Shapiro stresses the need to use measurements which reduce the subjective part of clinical decision making. He next delineates three attributes of objective information. It is documentable, specific and quantifiable.

The author next points out that use of the term "respiratory failure" as traditionally applied has been poorly defined and is overly broad in its application to clinical situations. It is neither specific nor quantitative. Shapiro then proceeds to show how correct evaluations of arterial blood gases can make this diagnosis objective by documenting primary oxygenation, ventilation or metabolic acid-base disturbances.

He follows with a discussion of the normal values of arterial blood gases. This discussion begins with the presentation of some basic statistical concepts. These concepts include the ideas of multiple manners of describing the central point in a collection of data, ways for describing the distribution of the data around the central points, and the shape of that distribution. From this discussion he moves to discussion of clinical significance, acceptable range and laboratory normal range.

The discussion then moves to the relationships between the variables in blood gases and acid-base balance. This portion of the chapter includes the relationships between:

P_aCO_2 and pH
P_aCO_2 and plasma HCO_3^-
$\dot{V}_E$ and $\dot{V}_A$
F_IO_2 and P_aO_2
S_aO_2 and P_aO_2

Additionally, Shapiro writes about the relationships between base buffers and pH. He states that under normal conditions the extremely effective buffering system in the body can moderate significantly large changes in acid content allowing little change in pH (free $[H^+]$). Shapiro contends that the degree of buffer deviation from normal can be calculated and is called *base excess* or *base deficit*. He also states that this can be calculated independent of PCO_2 compensation changes.

The direction and extent of the base excess/deficit depends on the difference between the predicted respiratory pH and the actual pH. Correction of base deficit should take place under set guidelines. This is done by administering $NaHCO_3$ IV. The following rules normally apply:

- Don't correct base deficits ↓ 10 mMol/L.
- Don't treat pH > 7.20 unless CV instability exists.
- Give only 50% of the correcting dose at a time.
- Check ABGs 5 minutes after $NaHCO_3$ administration.

Key Points

➢ Clinical judgements are sometimes made based on numerous observations, tests and measurements which vary in their objectivity, quantifiability and accuracy.

- These broad, ill-defined and poorly delineated diagnoses neither specify nor quantify the pathophysiology.
- Respiratory failure is an example of such a non-specific judgement.
- Diagnostic tests and the associated clinical judgements should be documentable, specific and quantifiable.
- Arterial blood gases provide documented, specific, quantified and repeatable measurements of respiratory failure.
- Blood gases allow differentation between primary oxygenation deficiencies, primary ventilation deficiencies and primary metabolic acid-base deficiencies.
- Individual differences within a species' biological functions tend to be distributed equally (symmetrically) around the arithmetic mean (average).
- When the frequency of occurrence of biological data are plotted, they are shaped like a bell (normal) curve.
- The area under the bell curve represents the population of all possible values within the boundaries of the curve.
- That portion of the area under the curve which represents the values of 33% of the data on either side of the mean (average) is one standard deviation (1 SD) (X =/– 33% of data).
- 2 SD = 95% of data; 3 SD = 99% of data. (Note: In statistics we say population instead of data; e.g., 2 SD = 95% of the population.)
- At 2 SD we can be 95% sure that the data we see is due to the factors governing the measured value, not chance. This is known as the (or a) 95% confidence level. (This means that there is a 2.5% chance that the real value is higher and a 2.5% chance that the real value is lower than those within the 2 SD range.)
- Normal ranges are determined by computing the means and standard deviations for large series of measurements from suitable populations. Normal ranges are reported as 1 or 2 SD distributions around the mean value for all measurements.
- Small variations from normal ranges in arterial blood gases are seldom of clinical significance even in the unstable patient.
- Acceptable ranges generally are based on clinical judgements developed by experience over time. They allow for the small variations outside the normal range.
- pH is primarily the result of the plasma bicarbonate - carbonic acid relationship.
- Although not entirely linear within clinical ranges, pH and P_aCO_2 are inversely related.
- From a P_aCO_2 of 40 mmHg, each 20 mmHg increase results in a 0.10 decrease in pH units (P_aCO_2 ↑ from 40 mmHg to 60 mmHg; pH ↓ from 7.40 to 7.30).
- From a P_aCO_2 of 40 mmHg, each 10 mmHg decrease results in a 0.10 increase in pH units (P_aCO_2 ↓ from 40 mmHg to 30 mmHg; pH ↑ from 7.40 to 7.50).
- Starting with a pH of 7.40, P_aCO_2 of 40 mmHg, and HCO_3^- of 24 mMol/L:
  Each 10 mmHg ↑ in P_aCO_2 increases HCO_3^- by 1 mMol/L.
  Each 10 mmHg ↓ in P_aCO_2 decreases HCO_3^- by 21 mMol/L.
- (Predicted HCO_3^-) – (actual HCO_3^-) = metabolic component.
- Total ventilation ($\dot{V}_E$) = alveolar ventilation ($\dot{V}_A$) + deadspace ventilation ($\dot{V}_D$): $\dot{V}_E = \dot{V}_A + \dot{V}_D$.
- Deadspace ventilation ($\dot{V}_D$) has two divisions, physiologic deadspace (V_{Dphys}) and anatomical deadspace (V_{Danat}): $\dot{V}_D = V_{Dphys} + V_{Danat}$.
- During exercise, in the normal individual, $\dot{V}_E$ increases but V_{Dphys} remains relatively constant, and V_{Danat} may decrease relative to the increase in $\dot{V}_E$ or may remain unchanged. Therefore $\dot{V}_A$ increases.
- Adequate cardiopulmonary reserves allow for offsetting changes in perfusion or ventilation should the other organ system become moderately compromised.
- Patients with increased MV with higher than predicted P_aCO_2 have either significantly increased deadspace ventilation or increased CO_2 production or a combination of both.
- Patients with decreased $\dot{V}_A$ with higher than predicted P_aCO_2 and lower than expected MV have either significantly increased deadspace ventilation or increased CO_2 production or a combination of both.
- Minute ventilation to P_aCO_2 disparity suggests deadspace producing pathology.
- The normal alveolar to arterial (A-a) gradient is 4 mmHg in a healthy individual breathing room air at sea level.
- Hypoxemia is defined as a P_aO_2 less than 80 mmHg.
- Normal P_aO_2 is somewhat age-dependent at the extremes of the age ranges. Normal P_aO_2 in newborns is 40 to 70 mmHg; for persons over 60 P_aO_2 is 80 mmHg – 1 mmHg (age – 60).
- Each 0.1 (10%) increase in F_IO_2 increases P_aO_2 by 75 mmHg or P_aO_2 by 50 mmHg.
- Desired % $F_IO_2 \times 5$ = predicted P_aO_2.

- If actual P_aO_2 is less than predicted P_aO_2, assume patient will be hypoxemic breathing room air.
- The blood's ability to moderate the effects of large changes in acid (free H^+) concentration depends on its base buffer system.
- The variation from normal base buffer content is called base excess or base deficit depending on the direction of change.
- The greater the variation from normal, the larger the pH change for any given $[H^+]$ change.
- A base excess/deficit of +/– 5 mMol/L of normal is considered to be within the acceptable range.
- A base excess/deficit of +/– 10 mMol/L of normal is considered to be a significant acid-base imbalance.
- From an assumed baseline of pH of 7.40 and P_aCO_2 of 40 mmHg, an acute rise of 10 mmHg in P_aCO_2 results in a pH decrease of 0.05 units (P_aCO_2 changes from 40 mmHg to 50 mmHg; pH changes from 7.40 to 7.35).
- From an assumed baseline of pH of 7.40 and P_aCO_2 of 40 mmHg, an acute fall of 10 mmHg in P_aCO_2 results in a pH rise of 0.10 units (P_aCO_2 changes from 40 mmHg to 30 mmHg; pH changes from 7.40 to 7.50).
- Predicted respiratory pH =

  If $P_aCO_2 > 40$ [(measured P_aCO_2 – 40)/100]/2 – 7.40

  If $P_aCO_2 < 40$ [(40 – measured P_aCO_2) /100] + 7.40
- The metabolic component of base buffer excess/deficit is the difference between the predicted respiratory pH and the measured pH.
- Metabolic pH change =

  [100(measured pH – Predicted respiratory pH)]2/3 $\simeq$ base excess/deficit
- Base deficits should be only 50% corrected on the first administration.
- Arterial pH > 7.20 should not be treated unless CV instability is present.
- Base deficits < 10 mMol/L should not be routinely treated.

Formulas

Predicted pH (acute)

Assume: initial arterial P_aCO_2 = 40 mmHg
initial arterial pH = 7.40

For observed P_aCO_2 > 40 mmHg
Predicted pH = (mmHg ↑ P_aCO_2 × 0.005) – 7.40
Note: pH ↓ 0.10 for every 20 mmHg ↑ in P_aCO_2

or

For observed P_aCO_2 < 40 mmHg
Predicted pH = (mmHg ↓ P_aCO_2 /100) + 7.40
Note: pH ↑ 0.10 for each 10 mmHg ↓ in P_aCO_2

Predicted Plasma Bicarbonate (HCO_3^-)

Assume: initial arterial P_aCO_2 = 40 mmHg
initial arterial pH = 7.40
initial plasma bicarbonate = 24 mMol/L

For observed P_aCO_2 > 40 mmHg
Predicted plasma HCO_3^- mMol/L = 24 + 0.1 (observed P_aCO_2 – 40)
Note: HCO_3^- ↑s by 1 mMol/L for each 10 mmHg ↑ in CO_2

or

For observed P_aCO_2 < 40 mmHg
Predicted plasma HCO_3^- mMol/L = 24 – 0.2 (observed P_aCO_2 – 40)
Note: HCO_3^- ↓s by 2 mMol/L for each 10 mmHg ↓ in P_aCO_2

Minute Ventilation to P_aCO_2 Disparity

$$P_aCO_2 \text{ disp} = \frac{\text{change in } P_aCO_2 \text{ mmHg}}{\text{change in MV L}}$$

A-a Oxygen Gradient

A-a Oxygen Gradient = $P_AO_2 - P_aO_2$

P_AO_2 Determination

$P_AO_2 = [F_IO_2 (P_B - PH_2O)] - P_aCO_2$
where PH_2O = 47 mmHg (assuming normal body temperature)

Age Compensation for P_aO_2

For persons 60-90 years of age breathing room air predicted P_aO_2 mmHg = 80 mmHg – (patient's age – 60)

Predicted P_aO_2 when Administering O_2 Enriched Gas

Predicted P_aO_2 = (Change in F_IO_2 % × 50) + initial P_aO_2

Minimal acceptable P_aO_2 = (F_IO_2 % × 5) or (F_IO_2 × 500)

Predicted Respiratory pH

if P_aCO_2 obs ↑ 40 mmHg
7.40 – {[(P_aCO_2 obs – 40 mmHg)/2] × 0.01} = pred pH

if P_aCO_2 obs ↓ 40 mmHg
7.40 + [(40 mmHg – P_aCO_2 obs) × 0.01] = pred pH

Metabolic Component of pH

$$\text{Base excess/deficit} = \frac{2\,[(\text{pH obs} - \text{pH pred}) \times 0.015]}{3}$$

Note: pH pred = predicted Respiratory pH from previous formula

if predicted pH ↑ pH observed – base deficit

if predicted pH ↓ pH observed – base excess

Base Deficit Correction

Base Deficit*/2 = Initial $NaHCO_3$ correcting dose
* from previous formula

Tables and Figures

ABG Variable	*Units*	*Mean*	*1 SD*	*2 SD*	*"Acceptable"*
pH	—	7.40	7.38 - 7.42	7.35 - 7.45	7.33 - 7.48
P_aCO_2	mmHg	40	38 - 42	35 - 45	33 - 47
P_aO_2	mmHg	90	95 - 98	80 - 100	75 - 100
HCO_3^-	mMol/L	24	23 - 25	22 - 26	20 - 28

Table 1: Normal values for arterial blood gas values.

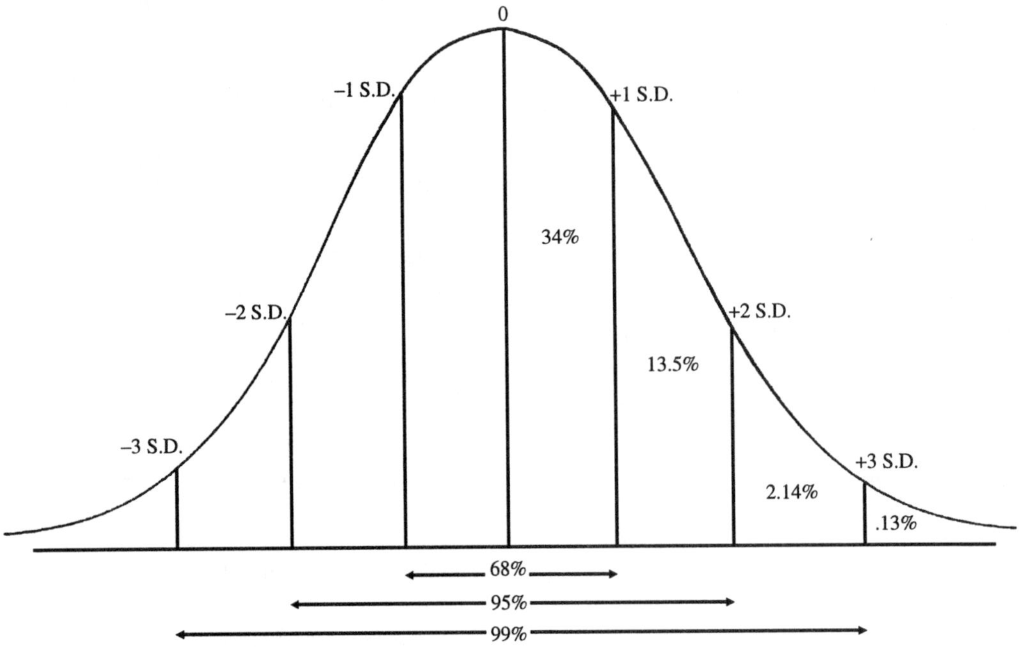

Figure 1: Normal bell curve with 1, 2 and 3 standard deviations illustrated.

Problems

Select and mark the best answer.

1. Identify, by number sequence, the mean values for arterial blood gases.

	pH	P_aCO_2	P_aO_2	HCO_3^-
I.	7.40	48	86	30
II.	7.49	45	59	24
III.	7.32	40	72	20
IV.	7.25	37	105	18
V.	7.53	31	90	35

	pH	P_aCO_2	P_aO_2	HCO_3^-
a.	II	IV	III	V
b.	I	III	V	II
c.	I	I	IV	IV
d.	II	IV	V	I
e.	V	III	II	III

2. Given F_IO_2 0.70, P_aO_2 157 and P_B 755 mmHg, which of the following is the calculated A-a oxygen gradient if the patient's temperature is normal (to nearest whole number)?
   a. 529 mmHg
   b. 432 mmHg
   c. 105 mmHg
   d. 117 mmHg
   e. 339 mmHg

3. An objective and definitive clinical test has all of the following features except
   a. it is specific.
   b. it is documentable.
   c. it is quantifiable.
   d. it is immediate.
   e. Both a and b are correct.

4. Biological data tends to be symmetrically distributed around the most common (most frequently observed) value. Symmetrical distribution means that when the frequency of all of the observed values are plotted on a graph the result is
   a. a bell-shaped curve.
   b. a downward sloping line.
   c. an upward sloping line.
   d. an S-shaped curve.
   e. straight parallel lines.

5. *Normal range* refers to the symmetrical frequency distribution of data which encompasses two standard deviations (2 SD) from the mean. What % of the total data falls within this range of values?
   a. 66%
   b. 75%
   c. 95%
   d. 99%
   e. 100%

6. Acceptable ranges of clinical values' "data"
   a. are generally larger than the normal range.
   b. recognize that small variations are seldom harmful.
   c. have proven to be both practical and dependable.
   d. All of the above are correct.
   e. Both a and b are correct.

7. Tommy Smith has had blood gases drawn and analyzed. Given the following data, calculate the predicted plasma bicarbonate (HCO_3^-): pH 7.40, P_aCO_2 30 mmHg.
   a. 30 mMol/L
   b. 28 mMol/L
   c. 26 mMol/L
   d. 24 mMol/L
   e. 22 mMol/L

8. For the above situation, assume that there was a question about the accuracy of the pH. Use the P_aCO_2 to predict the acute pH value.
   a. 7.35
   b. 7.50
   c. 7.45
   d. 7.40
   e. 7.55

9. If the observed P_aCO_2 in problems 7 and 8 had been 45 mmHg, what would the predicted acute pH be?
   a. 7.425
   b. 7.525
   c. 7.375
   d. 7.400
   e. 7.500

10. Which of the following statements is true in view of the deep breathing caused by exercising?
    a. V_{Dphys} increases with increased MV.
    b. Lung perfusion decreases as MV increases.
    c. V_{Danat} increases in proportion to MV as MV increases.
    d. V_{Danat} decreases in proportion to MV as MV increases.
    e. Both V_{Danat} and V_{Dphys} are unchanged with MV increases.

11. At or above which of the following P_aO_2 values would a 35-year-old male patient not be considered to be hypoxemic?
    a. 80 mmHg
    b. 70 mmHg
    c. 60 mmHg
    d. 75 mmHg
    e. 65 mmHg

12. Casey M. is a 72-year-old male admitted for a pre op workup due to an impending cholecystectomy. What is Casey's predicted P_aO_2 on room air? Assume that he has normal pulmonary function and physiology.
    a. 92 mmHg
    b. 85 mmHg
    c. 82 mmHg

d. 76 mmHg
e. 68 mmHg

13. If we increase % F_IO_2 by 10% at sea level, what P_aO_2 can we expect to see?
a. 47 mmHg
b. 76 mmHg
c. 50 mmHg
d. 21 mmHg
e. 10 mmHg

14. If the F_IO_2 is 0.45, what is the minimally acceptable P_aO_2 for that F_IO_2?
a. 130 mmHg
b. 175 mmHg
c. 200 mmHg
d. 225 mmHg
e. 300 mmHg

15. What degree of change in base excess/deficit in conjunction with an abnormal pH indicates a significant clinical acid-base balance change?
a. +/– 10 mMol/L
b. +/– 7 mMol/L
c. +/– 5 mMol/L
d. +/– 12 mMol/L
e. +/– 15 mMol/L

Answers to Problems

1. b: The mean or average normal values for the arterial blood gas variables are pH 7.40, P_aCO_2 40, P_aO_2 90, HCO_3^- 24.

2. e: The oxygen gradient (A-aDO_2) equals the P_AO_2 – the P_aO_2. P_AO_2 equals $(P_B - PH_2O) \times F_IO_2$. PH_2O is a temperature related variable and equals 47 mmHg at body temperature. Thus:
Given: $P_B = 755$ mmHg, $PH_2O = 47$ mmHg
$P_aO_2 = 157$ mmHg, $F_IO_2 = 0.70$
and
$$A\text{-}aDO_2 = [(P_B - PH_2O) \times F_IO_2] - P_aO_2$$
substituting:
$$A\text{-}aDO_2 = [(755 - 47) \times 0.70] - 157$$
$$= (708 \times 0.70) - 157$$
$$= 495.6 - 157$$
$$= 338.6$$
$$\simeq 339$$

3. d: The characteristics of specific (ability to locate the origin of damage/disorder), documentable (the ability to provide an objective record of a value or event) and quantifiable (the attribute of measuring in a repeatable and recordable manner) all lead to objective and definitive clinical testing. While speed is important, it does not lead to objectivity.

4. a: A bell-shaped curve results from a symmetrical distribution of the frequency of observed values. This occurs for three reasons: first, there tends to be a value which occurs more often than other values (Central Tendency). Second, other values tend to spread around the most common value(s) (Distributive Tendency). That is, each observation is equally likely to occur at a frequency higher or lower than the frequency at which the most common value occurs. Third, the further from the midpoint value, the lower the frequency of occurrence.

5. c: The symmetrical frequency distribution means that there are an equal number of values on either side of the midpoint (mean). 2 SD indicates that it is likely that 95% (47.5% on each side of the mean) of all of the observations occur and can be accounted for within this portion of the bell (normal) curve. This is also called the 95% confidence level.

6. d: Acceptable ranges exist due to experience and custom. They recognize that illness and injury cause small variations in the normal ranges of physiologic variables and individual response. These variations are not likely to be harmful but "push the edge" of the data curve's normal range, resulting in a larger range of acceptable values. This is practical and dependable because it prevents "overtreatment," and because it derives from long, successful clinical practices.

7. e: HCO_3^- decreases by 2 mMol/L for each 10 mmHg increase in P_aCO_2.
If "normal" $HCO_3^- = 24$ mMol/L
and
P_aCO_2 difference = observed P_aCO_2 – "normal" P_aCO_2
P_aCO_2 difference = 30 mmHg – 40 mmHg = –10 mmHg
and
–10 mmHg P_aCO_2 = –2 mMol/L HCO_3^-
then
24 mMol/L – 2 mMol/L HCO_3^- = 22 mMol/L

8. b: An increase of 0.10 units in pH occurs with each 10 mmHg decrease in P_aCO_2 (the blood becomes more alkalotic).
If "normal" P_aCO_2 = 40 mmHg
and
P_aCO_2 difference = observed P_aCO_2 – "normal" P_aCO_2
P_aCO_2 difference = 30 mmHg – 40 mmHg = –10 mmHg
and
–10 mmHg P_aCO_2 = + 0.10 pH units
then
predicted acute pH = initial pH + 0.10 =
7.40 + 0.10 = 7.50

9. c: For each 20 mmHg increase in P_aCO_2, pH will decrease by 0.10 units (↑ acidosis).
If "normal" P_aCO_2 = 40 mmHg
and

P_aCO_2 difference = observed P_aCO_2 – "normal" P_aCO_2

P_aCO_2 difference = 45 mmHg – 40 mmHg = 5 mmHg
and
20 mmHg increase in P_aCO_2 = 10 pH unit decrease
then
5 mmHg P_aCO_2 = –0.025 pH units
therefore
predicted acute pH = 7.40 – 0.025 = 7.375

10. d: V_{Danat} is a relatively fixed volume varying only by the elastic stretch caused by decreasing interthoracic pressures during inspiration. Therefore, as MV increases due to deeper breathing, the proportion of ventilation devoted to V_{Danat} remains relatively constant. V_{Dphys} decreases in most cases while pulmonary perfusion will increase under the exercise load. The net result is to increase V_{alv}, increasing gas exchange.

11. a: Arterial PO_2 of less than 80 mmHg is considered to indicate hypoxemia. An exception to the rule exists for both the older adult (above age 60) and the newborn.

12. e: For persons over age 60, normal P_aO_2 decreases (from the low "normal" of 80 mmHg by 1 mmHg for each year over 60). Therefore:

$$\begin{aligned} \text{Predicted } P_aO_2 \text{ for age} &= \text{Low normal } P_aO_2 - (\text{Patient age} - 60) \\ &= 80 \text{ mmHg} - (72 - 60) \\ &= 80 \text{ mmHg} - 12 \\ &= 68 \text{ mmHg} \end{aligned}$$

13. b:

$$\begin{aligned} P_IO_2 &= F_IO_2 \times P_B \\ &= .10 \times 760 \\ &= 76 \text{ mmHg} \end{aligned}$$

As the inspired gas descends the airway it is humidified at body temperature to saturation (PH_2O = 47 mmHg) and mixes with the endtidal CO_2 (PCO_2 = 40). The P_AO_2 increase has diminished, due to Dalton's Law.

$$\begin{aligned} P_AO_2 &= F_IO_2 \times [(P_B - PH_2O) - P_ACO_2] \\ &= 0.10 \times [(760 - 47) - 40] \\ &= 0.10 \times (713 - 40) \\ &= 0.10 \times 673 \\ &= 67.3 \end{aligned}$$

14. d: A good method for determining the lowest expected acceptable P_aO_2 which will result from a change in F_IO_2 is to multiply the desired F_IO_2 by 500.

$F_IO_2 \times 500$ = minimally acceptable P_aO_2

$0.45 \times 500 = 225$ mmHg

15. a: Changes of +/– 10 mMol/L are severe. This is especially true if pH changes are also evident indicating a potential failure of the acid-base buffer system. These conditions are clinically significant and should be acted upon promptly.

Case Study

Sara Z. is a 72-year-old white woman who presents to the ER with a chief complaint of acute onset SOB. The patient was well until 48 hours ago when she began to "have trouble catching my breath."

Past Medical History:
Multiple admissions over the last 3 years for:
Pneumonia × 4 of 1-3 weeks' duration
? CHF × 2 (borderline)
Fever of unknown origin × 1
Chronic gastric reflux × 3

Current Meds:
digitalis
8 oz. H_2O with 1 tbls $NaHCO_3$ QID

Social History:
Widowed × 6 years
ETOH - 1 shot bourbon QD at HS
Tobacco - 1 pack/day 18 yrs, quit 2 years ago

Physical Exam:
Neuro: Alert; oriented × 3
PERRLA
PNS intact and functional
CNS intact and functional
Chest:
Heart - Mild tachycardia, rate = 112/min
Slight ST depression in V2
Occasional long QRS with ↓ P waves
Muffled 2nd sounds
Lungs - A decreased inspiratory sounds in bases bilaterally. Expiratory rhonchi noted in R middle and lower lobes, L lower lobe ↓ to silent. Cough loose, non-productive.
P Dullness noted over R and L bases.
O Decreased movement of basilar ribs. ↑ AP diameter, slight nasal flaring at end inspiration. Right lateral chest wall tender with guarding. Cyanosis noted in mucus membranes.

GI: ? hyperacidity - gastric reflux. Not tender.

Gyn: Not contributory

Vital signs:
P = 112 bpm
R = 24/min, shallow
BP = 136/96
T = 37.5 C (oral)

Laboratory:
ABGs: pH 7.46, P_aO_2 60 mmHg, P_aCO_2 = 46 mmHg, HCO_3^- = 30 mMol/L, F_IO_2 = 0.21

CXR: Consolidation in both lower lobes. Right middle lobe shows evidence of pneumonia like processes. Air bronchogram is noted as are increased vascular markings. Right chest wall shows evidence of ? fracture of 9th and 10th ribs. IMP: Fx ribs, pneumonia, COPD.

Sputum: Blood tinged, (brown); viscid and stringy; culture not ready. Gram Stain unremarkable.

---

1. Is Sara's oxygenation normal for her age? What F_IO_2 is needed to increase her P_aO_2 to 75 mmHg? What effect do her pneumonia and fractured ribs have on her oxygenation?

2. What is Sara's base excess/deficit? What is her predicted respiratory pH and her metabolic pH? What is causing the increase in HCO_3^-?

3. Given the patient's increased P_aCO_2 and increased HCO_3^-, what steps are appropriate to "normalize" the acid-base imbalance? How would you classify her acid-base status?

4. Does mechanical ventilation offer any benefits to this patient? What are they? In lieu of mechanical ventilation, what other therapies would be appropriate in this case?

Suggested Additional Readings

Mathews, PJ, Chapter 6 (Assessment of ventilation) in Wissing, DR, Conrad, SA and George, RB, *Critical Care for the Cardiopulmonary Practitioner*, Appleton & Lange, Inc., Norwalk, CT. In press; projected publication date April 1994.

Wheelock, P, "Using mathematics to evaluate respiratory function," *RT: The Journal for Respiratory Care Practitioners,* 1992, 5(2):42-5.

Wilson, RF, *Critical Care Manual*, 2nd edition, F.A. Davis, Inc., Philadelphia, PA, 1992, pp. 389-423.

Witkowski, AS, *Pulmonary Assessment: A Clinical Guide,* J.B. Lippincott, Philadelphia, PA, 1985, Chapters 5, 6 and 7.

CHAPTER 6

Clinical Approach to Interpretation

Objectives

After reading Chapter 6 and successfully completing this chapter of the workbook the student will be able to:

1. Cite three reasons why an orderly, simple and sensible method of ABG interpretation is useful.
2. Explain why a clinical approach to interpretation must deviate from the classical academic or physiologic nomenclature.
3. Differentiate between the traditional and the clinical view of CO_2 elimination.
4. Define alveolar ventilation.
5. Explain the alveolar ventilation - P_aCO_2 relationship.
6. Discuss the ability to assess CO_2 homeostasis as a clinical measurement.
7. Explain why respiratory acidosis and ventilatory failure are the same clinical entity.
8. Explain the relationship between work of breathing and cardiopulmonary homeostasis.
9. List the symptoms of detrimental WOB (acute respiratory distress).
10. Characterize respiratory acidosis in terms of P_aCO_2 status.
11. List the three broad circumstances that can lead to alveolar hyperventilation.
12. Define the following terms:

acute	hemoglobin saturation
alveolar hyperventilation	homeostasis
alveolar hypoventilation	left shift
alveolar ventilation	metabolic rate
arterial oxygen tension	nomenclature
chemoreceptor	obtunded
chronic	oxygen content
clinically oriented	oxyhemoglobin dissociation curve
clinically relevancy	oxyhemoglobin status
compensation	primary abnormality
diaphoresis	reliability
driving force (pressure)	respiratory center
efficiency	ventilatory failure
hemoglobin content	work of breathing (WOB)
hemoglobin-oxygen affinity	

13. Discuss the concept of chemoreceptors and respiratory centers.
14. Identify both the locations and functions of the chemoreceptors and the respiratory centers.
15. Identify and explain the one circumstance in which alveolar hyperventilation can be considered a form of respiratory failure.
16. Explain why ventilatory failure (respiratory acidosis) is always a form of respiratory failure.
17. State the two basic steps to be followed when considering blood gas data.
18. Differentiate between ventilatory and respiratory status.
19. Identify the best indicator of ventilatory function.
20. List and explain the three categories into which P_aCO_2 may be divided with respect to ventilatory status.
21. Identify the two primary sources of acid-base imbalance.
22. State the factors which determine various states of alveolar ventilation.
23. Given appropriate data, differentiate between metabolic acidemia and metabolic alkalemia.
24. Explain the difference between chronic and acute ventilatory failure.
25. Define and state the normal value and range for hemoglobin content.
26. Define *oxyhemoglobin saturation.*
27. Discuss the causes and effects of right and left shifts in the oxyhemoglobin dissociation curve.
28. Identify the reasons why P_aCO_2 is used as the standard for oxygenation status rather than the S_aO_2.
29. Discuss the concept of driving force.
30. Given the appropriate data, calculate the driving force in a system and indicate its vector (direction).
31. Explain why severe hypoxemia is a direct threat to cellular oxygenation.
32. Describe the levels of hypoxemia used in the new nomenclature.

Definitions

acute Of sudden onset (without warning), e.g., acute appendicitis.

alveolar hyperventilation Alveolar ventilation greater than that needed to maintain CO_2 balance (normal P_aCO_2). Shapiro's "Respiratory Alkalosis" ($P_aCO_2 <$ 35 mmHg).

alveolar hypoventilation Alveolar ventilation less than that needed to maintain CO_2 balance (normal P_aCO_2). Shapiro's "Respiratory Acidosis" ($P_aCO_2 > 44$ mmHg).

alveolar ventilation (V_{alv}) The part of total ventilation which takes part in gas exchange with the pulmonary blood flow.

arterial oxygen tension Pressure exerted by the dissolved O_2 in the arterial blood plasma (P_aO_2).

chemoreceptor Biological "sensors" in the aorta, carotid arteries and jugular veins which react to changes in concentration of specific chemical compounds or ions. Chemoreceptors are either "inhibitors" (stop processes) or "activators" (start processes).

chronic Long-lasting, in existence for an extended period of time, e.g., chronic back pain.

clinically oriented A practical, results-oriented method or procedure (what should be done vs. why it should be done).

clinically relevant The degree to which the procedure or information is useful or important in clinical practice.

compensation The counterbalancing of any defect in structure or function. In acid-base abnormalities, compensation is the process that attempts to restore the blood pH to normal. In respiratory acid-base disorders, compensation occurs through the renal system.

diaphoresis "Sweating," perspiring, loss of fluid (H_2O) through the sweat glands.

driving force (pressure) The pressure gradient which exists between two points in a system. Driving pressure has both magnitude and direction (vector). Driving force (pressure) = $P_{Hi} - P_{Lo}$.

efficiency The relative amount of energy (work) expended to produce a desired result or end product. High efficiency means low energy input for high output; low efficiency means high energy input for low output.

hemoglobin content (gm/dL) The amount of hemoglobin in 100 ml (1 decaliter) of blood (normal = > 12 gm/dL, normal range = 12-14 gm/dL).

hemoglobin - oxygen affinity The attraction of or propensity for oxygen to bind with (be carried by) the heme molecule in the red blood cell. O_2 saturation is an indicator of this affinity. P_{50} is the most sensitive common indicator of affinity changes.

hemoglobin saturation (S_aO_2) See oxyhemoglobin status.

homeostasis The tendency of the body to maintain the stability of its chemical, physical and electromechanical systems in a state of dynamic balance. It involves a continuous process of adaptation and change in response to internal and external environmental factors.

left shift The curve shifts to the left, towards the Y axis, indicating an increase in hemoglobin's affinity for oxygen at a given P_aO_2.

metabolic rate The speed at which O_2 is utilized and CO_2 and H_2O are produced by energy production mechanisms in the cells.

nomenclature A system of naming, labeling or classifying items or conditions.

obtunded Insensitive to pain or sensation; unconscious.

oxygen content The total amount of oxygen, expressed in ml/dL, being carried in the blood, both combined with hemoglobin and dissolved in the plasma.

oxyhemoglobin dissociation curve A graphic representation of the relationship between oxygen saturation and P_aO_2.

oxyhemoglobin status (oxyhemoglobin saturation [S_aO_2]) A measure of the percent of hemoglobin molecules in the arterial blood which are saturated with (bound to) oxygen, i.e., how much oxygenated Hb is bound vs. how much there could be.

primary abnormality The initial or major cause of a physical, pathological or physiologic imbalance.

reliability The ability to give the correct answer and do so each time the same measurement is made under the same conditions.

respiratory center Chemo and proprio (pressure) receptors located in the brain stem (medulla oblongata) which control the rate and depth of ventilation (inspiratory, expiratory and pneumotaxic centers).

right shift The curve shifts to the right, away from the Y axis, indicating a decreased affinity (attraction) for oxygen by the hemoglobin at a given P_aO_2.

ventilatory failure The failure or inability of the pulmonary system to meet the metabolic demand for CO_2 elimination in an efficient and effective manner.

work of breathing (WOB) Energy cost of breathing; how much energy is needed to move a given volume of gas through the ventilatory process.

Introduction

In this chapter Shapiro develops and discusses a method to be used as a clinically valid interpretation system for arterial blood gases. His method is said to be reliable, simple and sensible. The method identifies the primary physiologic abnormalities, helps to identify the proper therapy, and allows gathering of information to guide that therapy.

He begins by pointing out that the terms developed for traditional, academic and physiologic studies of acid-base balance are of limited clinical use as interpretation tools. Shapiro next develops the concept of ventilatory failure as a clinically relevant attempt to maintain CO_2 homeostasis. This is based on the attempt of the body to correct CO_2 imbalance and to maintain a normal range of pH. Shapiro stresses that only alveolar ventilation can eliminate CO_2 quickly and efficiently. Ventilatory failure, he states, is related only to ventilation, not to oxygenation, and is assessed in terms of CO_2 homeostasis.

In that CO_2 homeostasis is a balance between the production of CO_2 as a byproduct of metabolic processes and the elimination of CO_2 by excretion in the exhaled breath, *ventilatory failure* is defined as "... the condition in which the pulmonary system is unable to meet the metabolic demands of the body in relation to CO_2 homeostasis." Ventilatory failure is the same clinical entity commonly described as respiratory acidosis. The causes of this condition are discussed next with special emphasis put on the role of work of breathing (WOB). Shapiro states that although normal WOB is beneficial to cardiopulmonary homeostasis, extreme WOB is represented by acute respiratory distress. In respiratory alkalosis, P_aCO_2 is lower than normal due to alveolar hyperventilation, i.e., alveolar ventilation which exceeds the level necessary to maintain P_aCO_2 at normal levels. Alveolar hyperventilation occurs due to stimulation of peripheral and central chemoreceptors by increased PCO_2 and by stimulation of the respiratory centers in the brain by altered pH, PCO_2 and PO_2.

Presenting a structured approach, Shapiro provides a two-step method for arterial blood gas interpretation. First, assess ventilatory status. Second, assess oxygenation (P_aO_2/S_aO_2) status. Shapiro states that the "normal" P_aCO_2 falls between 36 and 44 mmHg. Alveolar hyperventilation is evidenced by $P_aCO_2 <= 35$ mmHg. Alveolar hypoventilation, on the other hand, is indicated by $P_aCO_2 = > 45$ mmHg. By also assessing the pH it can be determined whether the primary deficit is respiratory (pH > 7.40) or metabolic (pH < 7.40).

Shapiro next illustrates the determination of:

1. Alveolar hyperventilation and pH <= 7.35
   Alveolar hyperventilation (respiratory alkalosis)
   Acute alveolar hyperventilation
   Subacute alveolar hyperventilation
2. Alveolar hyperventilation and pH <= 7.35
   Completely compensated metabolic acidosis
   Partially compensated metabolic acidosis
3. Normal ventilation (P_aCO_2 = 36-44 mmHg)
   Metabolic alkalemia (pH ↑ 7.44)
   Metabolic acidemia (pH ↓ 7.36)
4. Ventilatory failure (P_aCO_2 > 45; pH variable)
   Partially compensated metabolic acidosis
   Chronic ventilatory failure
   Acute ventilatory failure

Shapiro provides a series of practice exercises to aid in the comprehension of these interpretations. The exercises in this book are designed to supplement, not to substitute for, Shapiro's exercises.

Shapiro's discussion of assessment of arterial blood oxygenation begins by defining hemoglobin (Hb) content, oxyhemoglobin saturation and arterial oxygen tension. In the course of these discussions he explains the reasons that P_aO_2 rather than S_aO_2 is the primary and "gold" standard when assessing oxygenation. He also defines "clinically significant hypoxemia" as a $P_aO_2 < 60$ mmHg. He stresses that O_2 not be removed from patients, thus requiring that "probable" hypoxemia states be calculated (see Chapter 5). In conclusion he lists three criteria for categorizing levels of correction of hypoxemia:

1. Uncorrected hypoxemia $P_aO_2 < 60$ mmHg
2. Corrected hypoxemia $P_aO_2 > 60$ mmHg, < 100 mmHg
3. Excessively corrected hypoxemia $P_aO_2 > 100$ mmHg

Key Points

- The new method of interpretation will delineate the primary life-threatening physiologic abnormality.
- The method will help determine appropriate cardiopulmonary supportive therapy.
- It will also allow measurements which can guide therapy.
- Rather than viewing CO_2 excretion in terms of respiratory acid-base balance where CO_2 retention is associated with accumulation of free H^+ ions, from a clinical viewpoint CO_2 accumulation is seen as the failure of the pulmonary system to maintain CO_2 homeostasis.
- The clinical relevance of respiratory acid-base imbalance is its role in correcting the mechanisms of CO_2 elimination.
- Alveolar ventilation is the portion of tidal volume which engages in exchange of CO_2 and O_2 with the pulmonary capillary blood.
- Arterial PCO_2 is a direct reflection of the adequacy of CO_2 exchange.
- Regardless of the causal pathology, the primary clinical concern with CO_2 accumulation is the pulmonary system's inability to excrete CO_2.
- Ventilatory failure is an expression of the efficiency of CO_2 elimination.

- Respiratory failure includes both ventilatory failure (increased CO_2) and oxygenation failure (decreased O_2).
- Metabolic rate determines CO_2 production.
- It is assumed that P_aCO_2 is in equilibrium with P_ACO_2.
- P_aCO_2 reflects the match between CO_2 production (metabolism) and CO_2 elimination (ventilation).
- When CO_2 elimination by the alveolar ventilation matches CO_2 production, P_aCO_2 is normal.
- Ventilatory failure is the condition in which the pulmonary system is unable to meet the metabolic demands of the body in relation to CO_2 homeostasis.
- A diagnosis of ventilatory failure can be made only by means of arterial blood gas analysis.
- Ventilatory failure is diagnosed separately from arterial oxygenation status.
- Ventilatory failure is the same condition as respiratory acidosis.
- Respiratory acidosis is a reflection of a clinical abnormality which must be treated as a deficit in ventilation.
- Diseases which affect the efficiency or capability of CO_2 elimination may lead to ventilatory failure.
- Appropriate levels of WOB ensure proper levels of alveolar ventilation and maintain pulmonary perfusion and cardiac function by increasing venous return.
- Within the limits of cardiopulmonary reserves, normal WOB is beneficial to maintenance of cardiopulmonary homeostasis.
- WOB above the limits of cardiopulmonary reserves results in deterioration of cardiopulmonary function.
- Signs and symptoms of detrimental levels of WOB include tachycardia, tachypnea, dyspnea, intercostal retractions, hypertension, accessory muscle use, diaphoresis, and changes in mental status.
- Respiratory alkalosis is a clinical indicator that alveolar ventilation is greater than the metabolic demand to lower CO_2.
- Respiratory alkalosis is a state of alveolar hypoventilation resulting in a lower than normal P_aCO_2.
- Decreased alveolar PCO_2 results from either arterial hypoxemia (peripheral chemoreceptor stimulation) or metabolic acidosis (peripheral and/or central chemoreceptor stimulation or CNS respiratory center stimulation) or a combination of these.
- Alveolar hyperventilation can be considered a form of respiratory failure only if it results from an oxygen exchange failure.
- The system of interpretation used in this book is a structured approach.
- When interpreting any set of blood gases, you must assess both ventilation status (pH and P_aCO_2 homeostasis) and arterial oxygenation status.
- Arterial oxygenation status includes consideration of P_aO_2, S_aO_2 and O_2 content.
- P_aCO_2 <= 35 mmHg indicates hyperventilation.
- P_aCO_2 = 36-44 mmHg indicates normal ventilation.
- P_aCO_2 >= 45 mmHg indicates hypoventilation.
- Assessment of pH and P_aCO_2 permits decisions about whether the primary acid-base imbalance is respiratory (ventilatory) or metabolic.
- pH > 7.40, P_aCO_2 <= 35 mmHg = alveolar hyperventilation.
- pH > 7.40, P_aCO2 <= 35 mmHg = metabolic acidosis.
- pH >= 7.45, P_aCO_2 <= 35 mmHg = acute alveolar hyperventilation.
- pH = 7.40-7.44, P_aCO_2 <= 35 mmHg = chronic alveolar hyperventilation.
- pH = 7.45-7.50, P_aCO_2 <= 35 mmHg = sub-acute alveolar hyperventilation.
- pH = 7.36-7.40, P_aCO_2 <= 35 mmHg = completely compensated metabolic acidosis.
- pH <= 7.35, P_aCO_2 <= 35 mmHg = partially compensated metabolic acidosis.
- pH >= 7.45, P_aCO_2 = 36-44 mmHg = metabolic alkalemia.
- pH <= 7.35, P_aCO_2 = 36-44 mmHg = metabolic acidosis.
- pH >= 7.45, P_aCO_2 >= 45 mmHg = partially compensated metabolic alkalemia (may also mean acute or chronic ventilatory failure).
- pH = 7.36-7.44, P_aCO_2 >= 45 mmHg = chronic ventilatory failure.
- pH <= 7.35, P_aCO_2 >= 45 mmHg = acute ventilatory failure.
- P_aCO_2 and pH values must fall into one of seven abnormal categories, four ventilatory and three metabolic acid-base classes.
- Renal compensation is not clinically significant unless pH < 7.50, P_aCO_2 <= 30 mmHg.
- The renal system seldom compensates for respiratory alkalosis when pH < 7.45.

- Renal compensation takes about 24 hours to occur.
- pH <= indicates primary metabolic acidosis with pulmonary (ventilatory) compensation by hyperventilation.
- Normal hemoglobin (Hb) content is 12-14 gm/dL in adults.
- Hb levels > 8 gm/dL are enough to provide adequate O_2 carrying capacity in patients with good myocardial function.
- Oxyhemoglobin saturation (S_aO_2) is the best reflection of oxygen content because most of the oxygen in the blood is bound to hemoglobin.
- When normal P_aO_2 to S_aO_2 relationships are upset, a change in the hemoglobin - oxygen affinity has occurred.
- A decreased affinity causes a shift to the right in the oxyhemoglobin dissociation curve.
- A right shift indicates that the S_aO_2 is less than predicted for the observed P_aO_2.
- In the case of the right shifted curve, clinical judgements should be based on the S_aO_2, not on the P_aO_2.
- Arterial oxygen tension is the P_aO_2 and is accurate for values in the range of 30-200 mmHg.
- Arterial hypoxemia is a $P_aO_2 < 80$ mmHg breathing room air.
- Between S_aO_2 values of 90 and 95% there is no significant clinical improvement in O_2 delivery to the cells.
- $S_aO_2 = 90\% \simeq P_aO_2 = 60$ mmHg.
- Clinically significant hypoxemia results from $P_aO_2 <$ 60 mmHg.
- $P_aO_2 = 40$-60 mmHg (moderate hypoxemia) provides adequate tissue oxygenation given good cardiovascular and O_2 consumption performance.
- $P_aO_2 < 40$ mmHg (severe hypoxia) is a direct threat to tissue oxygenation.
- $P_aO_2 < 40$ mmHg results in decreased driving force across systemic cell walls.
- $P_aO_2 < 40$ mmHg = $S_aO_2 < 75\%$, thus increasing oxyhemoglobin affinity, causing a "tighter bond" between oxygen and the hemoglobin molecule and attracting more oxygen from solution into a "bound" state.
- Oxygen therapy should not be withheld or withdrawn to assess hypoxemia; instead use the prediction equations from Chapter 5 to determine the predicted values.
- $P_aO_2 <= 60$ mmHg with $F_IO_2 => 21\%$ = uncorrected hypoxemia.
- $P_aO_2 = 61$-100 mmHg with $F_IO_2 > 21\%$ = corrected hypoxemia.
- $P_aO_2 > 100$ mmHg with $F_IO_2 => 21\%$ = excessively corrected hypoxemia.
- If the observed P_aO_2 is greater than the minimal calculated P_aO_2, the patient may not be hypoxemic when breathing room air.
- Oxygen levels should be decreased and the results evaluated in a step-wise fashion.

Formulas

Alveolar Ventilation

Tidal Volume – (Physiological Deadspace + Anatomic Deadspace)

or

$$V_{alv} = V_T - (V_{Dphys} + V_{Danat})$$

Oxygen Content (O_2 Content)

Dissolved O_2 + Combined O_2

Driving Pressure (P_D)

Driving pressure = High Pressure – Low Pressure

or

$$P_D = P_{Hi} - P_{Lo}$$

Tables and Figures

P_aCO_2	Nomenclature
<= 35 mmHg	Alveolar hyperventilation (Respiratory acidosis)
36 - 44 mmHg	Normal alveolar ventilation
>= 45 mmHg	Alveolar hypoventilation (Respiratory alkalosis)

Table 1: Classification of P_aCO_2 levels.

P_aO_2	Nomenclature
< 60 mmHg	Uncorrected hypoxemia
60 - 100 mmHg	Corrected hypoxemia
> 100 mmHg	Excessively corrected hypoxemia

Table 2: Classification of P_aO_2 levels.

P_aCO_2	pH	Specific Classification	Common Nomenclature
< 35	> 7.45	Acute alveolar hyperventilation	Respiratory alkalosis
	7.40 - 7.44	Chronic alveolar hyperventilation	Respiratory alkalosis
	7.45 - 7.50	Sub-acute alveolar hyperventilation	Respiratory alkalosis
< 35	7.36 - 7.40	Completely compensated metabolic acidosis	Metabolic acidosis
	<= 7.35	Partially compensated metabolic acidosis	Metabolic acidosis
40 +	>= 7.45	—	Metabolic alkalemia
	<= 7.35	—	Metabolic acidemia
> 45	>= 7.45	Ventilatory failure, partially compensated metabolic alkalosis	Respiratory acidosis
	7.36 - 7.44	Chronic ventilatory failure	Respiratory acidosis
	<= 7.35	Acute ventilatory failure	Respiratory acidosis

Table 3: Classification of acid-base states.

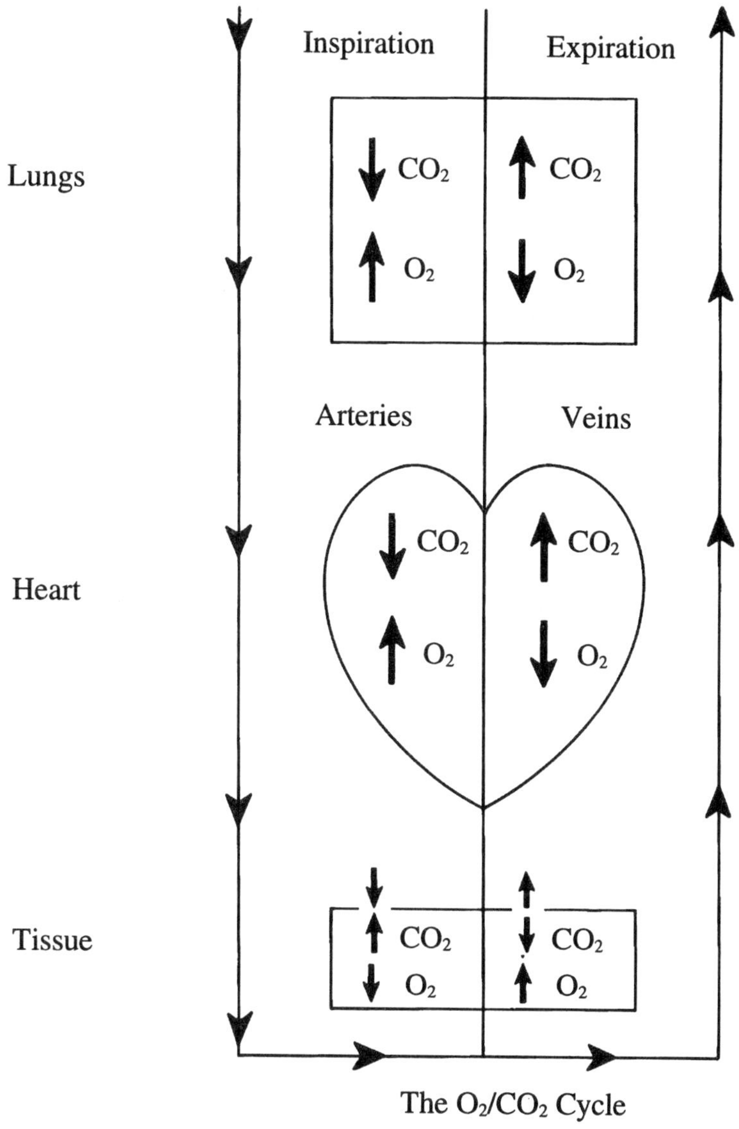

Figure 1: The O_2/CO_2 cycle.

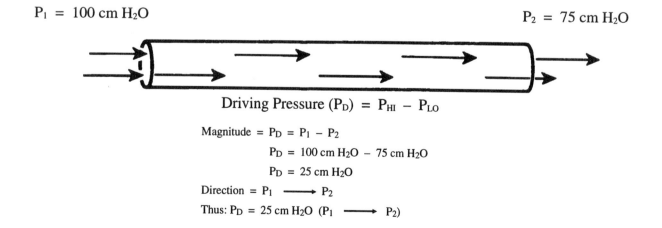

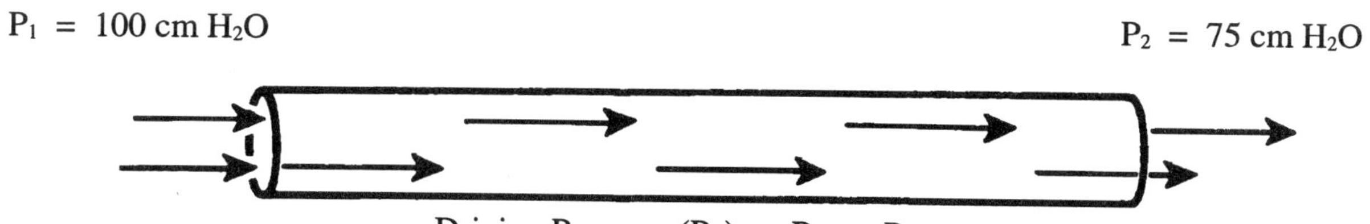

Driving Pressure (P_D) = $P_{HI} - P_{LO}$

Magnitude = $P_D = P_1 - P_2$

$P_D = 100 \text{ cm } H_2O - 75 \text{ cm } H_2O$

$P_D = 25 \text{ cm } H_2O$

Direction = $P_1 \longrightarrow P_2$

Thus: $P_D = 25 \text{ cm } H_2O \ (P_1 \longrightarrow P_2)$

Figure 2: Driving pressure (force).

Problems

Select and mark the best answer.

1. Which of the following is not used as part of the assessment of arterial oxygenation?
   a. Hemoglobin content
   b. P_aO_2
   c. S_aO_2
   d. pH
   e. Both a and d are correct.

2. Which of the following is true?
   a. The traditional academic view of CO_2 accumulation is that of a biochemical accumulation of free H^+ ions.
   b. The new nomenclature serves diagnostic purposes but does not guide therapeutic decisions.
   c. The new nomenclature takes the place of and is not compatible with the traditional system,
   d. Both the traditional and new nomenclature were based upon the ready clinical availability of arterial blood gas data.
   e. Both a and d are correct.

3. Which of the following is true regarding CO_2 homeostasis?
   a. CO_2 increases represent a failure of the pulmonary system to meet metabolic needs.
   b. The clinical relevance of acid-base balance is that it indicates the need for correction of the CO_2 elimination process.
   c. CO_2 exchange is dependent on adequate alveolar ventilation.
   d. P_aCO_2 is a direct reflection of the body's ability to use alveolar ventilation to control CO_2 homeostasis.

4. Alveolar ventilation is
   a. that part of the inspired gas volume which takes part in gas exchange.
   b. an indication of P_aCO_2 excess.
   c. found by estimating tidal volume and dividing by 2.
   d. tidal volume plus physiologic deadspace.
   e. physiologic plus anatomic deadspace.

5. Ventilatory failure encompasses all of the following except
   a. inability to maintain CO_2 homeostasis.
   b. it requires physiologic assessment of the pulmonary system.
   c. it requires assessment of the effectiveness of CO_2 removal.
   d. it is diagnosed by arterial blood gases.
   e. it requires assessment of oxygenation status.

6. Which of the following is a synonym for "ventilatory failure"?
   a. Respiratory distress syndrome
   b. Work of breathing
   c. Respiratory acidosis
   d. Lactic acidosis
   e. Metabolic acidosis

7. Work of breathing (WOB)
   a. increases as ventilatory failure improves.
   b. is the energy required to maintain ventilation.
   c. has little effect on cardiopulmonary homeostasis.
   d. decreases venous return and pulmonary perfusion.
   e. is independent of other influences on C-P balance.

8. Respiratory alkalosis
   a. describes a below normal P_aCO_2.
   b. results from alveolar hyperventilation.
   c. occurs when alveolar ventilation exceeds metabolic needs.
   d. All of the above are correct.
   e. Both a and b are correct.

9. Decreased alveolar CO_2 (P_ACO_2) occurs due to all of the following except
   a. arterial hypoxemia stimulating peripheral chemoreceptors.
   b. decreased alveolar ventilation.
   c. metabolic acidosis stimulating peripheral or central chemoreceptors.
   d. abnormal stimulation of brain stem respiratory centers.
   e. increased rate and/or depth of ventilation.

10. Interpretation of arterial blood gases requires two basic steps. These are
    I. Assessment of respiratory compliance
    II. Assessment of ventilatory status
    III. Assessment of arterial oxygenation
    IV. Assessment of work of breathing

    a. II and III
    b. I and II
    c. I and III
    d. II and IV
    e. I and IV

11. In order to diagnose the patient's primary acid-base abnormality, which of the following must be determined?
    a. P_aO_2 and P_aCO_2
    b. pH and P_aO_2
    c. pH and P_aCO_2
    d. P_aO_2 and S_aO_2
    e. S_aO_2 and P_aCO_2

12. Normal alveolar ventilation is indicated by
    a. P_aO_2 => 100 mmHg.
    b. pH = 7.35-7.45.
    c. % S_aO_2 = 95-100.
    d. HCO_3^- => 14 mMol/L.
    e. P_aCO_2 = 36-44 mmHg.

13. Which of the following represents chronic alveolar hyperventilation?
    a. pH 7.48, P_aCO_2 30 mmHg
    b. pH 7.42, P_aCO_2 33 mmHg
    c. pH 7.40, P_aCO_2 40 mmHg
    d. pH 7.50, P_aCO_2 20 mmHg
    e. pH 7.30, P_aCO_2 53 mmHg

14. Ventilatory failure is indicated by which of the following P_aCO_2s?
    a. 35 mmHg
    b. 42 mmHg
    c. 38 mmHg
    d. 48 mmHg
    e. 44 mmHg

15. Given the following data, calculate the driving force and direction (vector) of gas movement.
    Location: A B
    Pressure: 39 mmHg 52 mmHg

    a. 10 mmHg A —> B
    b. 91 mmHg A —> B
    c. 13 mmHg B —> A
    d. 1.5 mmHg B —> A
    e. 22 mmHg B —> A

Answers to Problems

1. d: pH does not play a major role in arterial oxygenation. Its effect is to cause mild right or left shifts of the oxyhemoglobin dissociation curve. On the other hand, the hemoglobin concentration, P_aO_2 and S_aO_2 are major determinants of oxygenation.

2. a: The traditional approach focused on pH $[H^+]$ and saw increased CO_2 as a byproduct of $[H^+]$ decrease. The new system sees CO_2 homeostasis as the driving force for pH balance. This view became viable only with the clinical availability of arterial blood gas measurements.

3. e: CO_2 homeostasis is a complex process involving metabolic production of CO_2 as a byproduct of cellular energy production and the elimination of CO_2 by the pulmonary system. Elimination or retention of CO_2 is the major method of pH stabilization in the body. The level of CO_2 is inversely related to the level of alveolar ventilation.

4. a: Alveolar ventilation – tidal volume – (physiologic deadspace + anatomical deadspace). It is the portion of the tidal volume which takes part in gas exchange in the lungs. Adequacy of alveolar ventilation is best assessed by arterial blood gas analysis.

5. e: Ventilatory failure is diagnosed by use of arterial blood gas data. Arterial blood gases are physiologic measures. Oxygenation is a separate issue and does not play a part in the diagnosis of ventilatory failure. The primary measures used to make the diagnosis of ventilatory failure are the pH and P_aCO_2. The diagnosis is made when blood gas analysis shows failure to maintain CO_2 homeostasis.

6. c: Ventilatory failure causes increased P_aCO_2 which results in an acidotic pH, thus the reference to respiratory acidosis. While increased WOB may result in ventilatory failure, the terms are not synonymous. Neither lactic acidosis nor metabolic acidosis are ventilatory problems; rather, they represent metabolic disorders. Respiratory distress syndrome may cause ventilatory failure but is not its only cause.

7. b: Work of breathing is an index of the amount of energy required to provide gas movement throughout the respiratory cycle. Although WOB is usually thought of as a single entity, in reality it consists of both inspiratory and expiratory components. WOB promotes pulmonary perfusion and venous return. WOB increases in many extra pulmonary diseases. Any condition which increases ventilatory failure also increases WOB.

8. d: Respiratory alkalosis is the traditional nomenclature which describes a low P_aCO_2 resulting from greater than normal levels of alveolar ventilation which exceeds the ventilation level necessary to reduce the CO_2, produced through metabolism, to normal levels.

9. b: Decreased alveolar ventilation will result in increased P_aCO_2. Increasing alveolar ventilation will decrease P_aCO_2. Alveolar ventilation is influenced by stimulation of the central and peripheral chemoreceptors and by stimulation or repression of the respiratory centers in the brain stem. There is, of course, a measure of voluntary control in the respiratory system. We can change the rate and depth of our respirations at will.

10. a: The primary values derived from arterial blood gas analysis are P_aCO_2, P_aO_2 and pH. Arterial P_aCO_2 is a measure of ventilation, while P_aO_2 is a measure of arterial oxygenation. WOB is not measured by means of ABGs. Compliance is an indicator of the pressure volume relationship within the pulmonary system but does not aid in interpreting ABGs.

11. c: Acid-base disorders are determined by the relationship between pH and P_aCO_2. The other factors listed are related to the oxygenation status of the patient.

12. e: Alveolar ventilation is responsible for controlling the level of CO_2. A P_aCO_2 between 36 and 44 mm Hg with a normal pH indicates a normal alveolar ventilation.

13. b: Chronic alveolar hyperventilation is characterized by pH values within the normal range and depressed P_aCO_2

values. The normal pH in the face of low CO_2 levels indicates that some compensatory metabolic mechanism is at work, most likely increased bicarbonate excretion or reduced conversion of metabolic acids.

14. d: Ventilatory failure is a condition under which normal pulmonary alveolar ventilation is unable to meet the demands of increased CO_2 production by the metabolism. The only abnormally high CO_2 indicated is 48 mmHg.

15. c: Driving force is the pressure differential across a system. When a pressure difference (gradient) exists, fluids (gas) flow from areas of high pressure to areas of low pressure in an attempt to equalize the pressure within the system. The driving force (pressure) is equal to the difference between the high and low pressures, and the direction of flow (vector) is from high to low pressure. In this example the flow vector is from B to A and the driving force (P_D) is 13 mmHg (52 – 39 mmHg).

Application Exercises

For the purposes of this section consider yourself the supervisor of the Blood Gas Laboratory at Anywhere Medical Center. An important part of your job is to do preliminary assessments of the arterial blood gases analyzed in your lab. The data is derived from the lab slips which contain only patient demographic data. No preliminary diagnosis is given, although the patient's ventilatory status may be indicated by checking Ventilator, Spontaneous, or Bagged on the request form.

The following blood gas reports are among those that were generated during the current shift. It is your task to analyze and interpret these results prior to releasing them to the requesting units.

1. Mrs. H J: 43-year-old female, spontaneous, F_IO_2 0.28, pH 7.32, P_aCO_2 34 mmHg, P_aO_2 104 mmHg, S_aO_2 99+%
   Interpretation:

2. Mr. L T: 35-year-old male, bagged, F_IO_2 0.98+, pH 7.04, P_aCO_2 15 mmHg, P_aO_2 304 mmHg, S_aO_2 99+%
   Interpretation:

3. Ms. B C: 26-year-old female, ventilated, F_IO_2 0.21, pH 7.54, P_aCO_2 55 mmHg, P_aO_2 71 mmHg, S_aO_2 81+%
   Interpretation:

4. Mrs. S V: 66-year-old female, ventilated, F_IO_2 0.40, pH 7.44, P_aCO_2 38 mmHg, P_aO_2 84 mmHg, S_aO_2 92+%
   Interpretation:

5. Mr. W F: 19-year-old male, spontaneous, F_IO_2 0.35, pH 7.44, P_aCO_2 38 mmHg, P_aO_2 84 mmHg, S_aO_2 92+%
   Interpretation:

6. Ms. A J: 34-year-old female, bagged, F_IO_2 0.90+, pH 7.22, P_aCO_2 58 mmHg, P_aO_2 184 mmHg, S_aO_2 97+%
   Interpretation:

7. Mr. H G: 89-year-old male, spontaneous, F_IO_2 0.21, pH 7.44, P_aCO_2 44 mmHg, P_aO_2 72 mmHg, S_aO_2 78+%
   Interpretation:

Answers to Application Exercises

1. Interpretation: Alveolar hyperventilation with excessively corrected hypoxemia. Possible acute partially compensated metabolic acidosis.
   Explanation: This patient is spontaneously hyperventilating (decreased P_aCO_2); her low pH indicates a marginal acidosis. The patient is receiving too much oxygen (increased P_aO_2). The problem is acute because the pH has not normalized and spontaneous hyperventilation cannot be maintained for long periods of time. The problem is metabolic because a decreased P_aCO_2 should result in a state of respiratory alkalosis.

2. Interpretation: Acute metabolic acidosis with hyperventilation. The patient is also excessively oxygenated.
   Explanation: This patient is in his mid-thirties and is being ventilated with a bag-valve unit. This suggests that the patient is in cardiac arrest or has markedly depressed respirations secondary to drug overdose or trauma. The extremely acidotic pH is suggestive of profound lactic acidosis secondary to hypoxemia and anaerobic metabolism. This again points to cardiac arrest. The patient is being manually ventilated at rates and/or volumes far in excess of his metabolic needs. Although increased P_aO_2 is indicated in cardiac resuscitation, levels above 150-200 mmHg have small additional benefit to the patient. Both decreases in F_IO_2 and the rate and/or volumes being provided by the manual resuscitator are warranted. Normalization of pH may require pharmaceutical intervention (THAM or Bicarb).

3. Interpretation: Ventilatory failure with moderate hypoxemia.
   Explanation: The patient's pH is appropriate for her P_aCO_2 (– 0.05 pH units per 10 mmHg increase in P_aCO_2); her P_aO_2 is low for her age, but not dangerously so. She is being mechanically ventilated at a minute volume which is inappropriately low to provide for adequate alveolar ventilation to meet her metabolic needs. Respiratory rate or tidal volume or both should be increased.

F_IO_2 should be increased to 24-26% to obtain a P_aO_2 in the 86-96 mmHg range.

4. Interpretation: Normal acid-base balance, corrected hypoxemia.
   Explanation: P_aCO_2 and pH are within normal limits. The patient is 66 years old; P_aO_2 decreases by about 1 mmHg per year of age over 60. Low normal P_aO_2 for persons of 60+ years of age is considered to be 80 mmHg (see Chapter 5).
   Predicted P_aO_2 = 80 mmHg − (age − 60)
   = 80 − (66 − 60)
   = 80 − 6
   = 74 mmHg

5. Interpretation: Ventilation is within normal limits; oxygenation status indicates corrected hypoxemia with moderate amounts of supplemental oxygen.
   Explanation: Although the pH to P_aCO_2 relationship is currently within normal (acceptable) range, there is a tendency toward metabolic alkalosis (pH is approaching 7.45+). There is a slight amount of hyperventilation present (P_aCO_2 is on the low side of normal). This needs to be followed. The patient's oxygenation is satisfactory but a bit low for his age.

6. Interpretation: Acute respiratory failure with both ventilatory failure and excessively corrected hypoxemia. Metabolic acidosis is also present.
   Explanation: The patient is being bagged at an insufficient rate or volume to meet her metabolic demands. There is also a component of metabolic acidosis (predicted respiratory pH = 7.31). The patient's P_aO_2 is excessively corrected, but this should not be a problem while the patient is being resuscitated. Correction of the F_IO_2 should be accomplished when the patient is stabilized.

7. Interpretation: Normal arterial blood gases.
   Explanation: All of the values measured or derived from these blood gases are normal for the patient's age. In fact, his P_aO_2 is markedly better than his predicted.
   Predicted P_aO_2 = 80 mmHg − (age − 60)
   = 80 − (89 − 60)
   = 80 − 19
   = 71 mmHg

Suggested Additional Readings

Levitzky, MG, *Pulmonary Physiology,* 3rd edition, McGraw-Hill, Inc., New York, NY, 1991, pp. 51-80.

Sproule, BJ, Lynne-Davies, P and King, EG, *Fundamentals of Respiratory Disease*, Churchill Livingstone, New York, NY, 1981, pp. 13-40.

Wilkins, RL and Dexter, JR, *Respiratory Disease: Principles of Patient Care,* F.A. Davis, Co., Philadelphia, PA, 1993, pp. 1-13.

CHAPTER 7

Assessment of the Lung as an Oxygenator

Objectives

After reading Chapter 7 and successfully completing this chapter of the workbook the student will be able to:

1. Define the term *intrapulmonary shunt.*
2. Define the divisions of intrapulmonary shunt and identify clinical conditions that cause each form of shunt.
3. Briefly explain the following shunt terms used in current medical literature:
   a. zero $\dot{V}/\dot{Q}$ or true shunt
   b. classic shunt
   c. physiologic shunt
4. Given a statement describing a physiologic variable used in the shunt and the Fick equations, match the variable to the statement it best describes.
5. Identify the ideal alveolar PO_2 at sea level.
6. Write the following equations:
   a. clinical shunt equation
   b. physiologic shunt equation
   c. Fick equation
   d. estimated shunt equation
7. Given a patient with acute pneumonia, briefly explain the single and combined effects of an elevated cardiac output and an increased F_IO_2 on the following:
   a. C_CO_2
   b. C_aO_2
   c. $C_{\bar{v}}O_2$
   d. a-v difference
   e. physiologic shunt
8. Differentiate between the $\dot{Q}_S/\dot{Q}_T$ and the $\dot{Q}_{sp}/\dot{Q}_T$.
9. Differentiate between the physiologic shunt equation and the clinical shunt equation.
10. Explain why the patient's body position should remain consistent when performing multiple shunt determinations.
11. Identify the steps used to ensure accuracy of the shunt measurement.
12. Identify the variables of the shunt equation derived directly from the patient's blood sample and those variables mathematically determined.
13. Identify when it is appropriate to use the estimated shunt equation in reflecting changes in the patient's physiologic shunt.
14. Identify the clinical circumstances in which the patient's $P_{(A\text{-}a)}O_2$ gives a satisfactory reflection of the amount of intrapulmonary shunting.
15. Given a list of gas exchange indices, identify the oxygen index that most closely reflects the critically ill patient's $\dot{Q}_{sp}/\dot{Q}_T$.
16. Identify the oxygen index that is more accurate in estimating the $\dot{Q}_S/\dot{Q}_T$.
17. Given hemodynamic and laboratory information, calculate the patient's physiologic shunt and estimated shunt.
18. Given hemodynamic and laboratory information, calculate the patient's oxygen consumption.

Definitions

anatomic shunt That portion of the cardiac output that enters the left side of the heart without traversing pulmonary capillaries.

capillary shunt That portion of the cardiac output that traverses the pulmonary capillaries but does not respire with alveolar gas.

classic shunt equation The calculation of the intrapulmonary shunt while the patient is breathing 100% inspired oxygen concentration. Originally believed to represent the true shunt.

estimated shunt equation An alternative equation to the physiologic shunt equation used in critically ill patients who do not have a pulmonary artery catheter in place and have adequate cardiovascular reserve.

Fick equation This equation shows the relationship between cardiac output, arteriovenous oxygen content and oxygen consumption.

intrapulmonary shunt That portion of the cardiac output entering the left side of the heart that does not have perfect gas exchange with perfect alveoli.

physiologic shunt The calculation of the intrapulmonary shunt at less than 100% inspired oxygen concentration. In a person breathing room air, this is the true measurement of the patient's normal shunt.

true shunt The arithmetic sum of the anatomic and capillary shunt. It is also referred to as zero $\dot{V}/\dot{Q}$.

venous admixture The blood that respires with alveolar units that contain less than the ideal oxygen tension. *Physiologic shunt* and *venous admixture* are synonymous terms.

Introduction

In Chapter 7 Shapiro discusses lung function relating to oxygenation of the pulmonary capillary blood. He explains the concept of intrapulmonary shunt and the different types of shunt an individual may develop: anatomic shunt, capillary shunt and venous admixture.

Everyone has a 2-5% anatomic shunt. A small percentage of cardiac output completely bypasses the lungs, resulting in this small amount of venous blood returning to the left heart and mixing with oxygenated blood from the lungs. The normal mixing of blood with two different oxygen saturations minimally reduces the oxygen content of the blood within the left heart. There are some pathologic conditions that can add to the individual's intrinsic anatomic shunt, such as tetralogy of fallot, tricuspid atresia, pulmonary atresia, persistent pulmonary hypertension of the newborn and transposition of the great vessels. Any one of these problems, in addition to the patient's intrinsic anatomic shunt, results in a significant effect on the individual's oxygenation.

Capillary shunt is secondary to a pulmonary problem and is not present in the normal lung. An individual with a disease or condition which impairs the oxygen exchange across the alveolar capillary membrane, such as atelectasis or severe pneumonia, has a capillary shunt.

Venous admixture, the last category of intrapulmonary shunt, does not meet the strict definition of shunt. The oxygenation defect in venous admixture is secondary to blood coming in contact with alveolar units that have reduced ventilation (low $\dot{V}/\dot{Q}$ units), not absent ventilation (zero $\dot{V}/\dot{Q}$ units). Therefore, the oxygen content of the blood flowing past low $\dot{V}/\dot{Q}$ units is higher than that of blood flowing past zero $\dot{V}/\dot{Q}$ units. However, the oxygenation may not be sufficient for the patient's metabolic needs.

The sum of the anatomic shunt and the capillary shunt is referred to as zero $\dot{V}/\dot{Q}$ or true shunt or, more simply, shunt. Venous admixture is referred to as $\dot{V}/\dot{Q}$, $\dot{V}/\dot{Q}$ inequity or shunt effect.

There are different expressions of shunt that should be clarified. $\dot{Q}_S/\dot{Q}_T$ is the representation of the zero $\dot{V}/\dot{Q}$. The patient is placed on 100% inspired oxygen concentration, and the patient's arterial and venous oxygen tension and saturation is measured. It is believed that by placing the patient on 100% oxygen, venous admixture no longer adds to the patient's shunt measurement.

$\dot{Q}_{sp}/\dot{Q}_T$ is called the physiologic shunt. It is measured when the patient is on less than 100% inspired oxygen concentration. Therefore, this intrapulmonary shunt measurement is a more realistic measurement of the function of the lung as a gas exchange organ in a person breathing room air. This measurement includes shunt and venous admixture. $\dot{Q}_{VA}/\dot{Q}_T$, known as venous admixture, is used interchangeably with $\dot{Q}_{sp}/\dot{Q}_T$. Some people object to using the term *physiologic* to refer to problems secondary to pathologic causes; e.g., pneumonia, emphysema and interstitial lung disease. Shapiro uses $\dot{Q}_{sp}/\dot{Q}_T$ to refer to the intrapulmonary shunt of a patient breathing less than 100% oxygen.

The shunt equation is measuring that portion of the patient's cardiac output that is not oxygenated by the lung. It compares the oxygen content of the shunted blood with the perfectly oxygenated blood of the nonshunted blood (Assumption: the blood is perfectly oxygenated by perfectly aerated alveolar units – the "ideal" lung.) Therefore, the shunt equation is a quantitative measurement of the oxygenation capability of the lung.

The initial reasoning steps in deriving the shunt equation are as follows:

1. If oxygen availability $= [\dot{Q}_T]\,[C_aO_2]$

2. If oxygen returned $= [\dot{Q}_T]\,[C_{\bar{v}}O_2]$

3. Then $VO_2 = ([\dot{Q}_T]\,[C_aO_2]) - ([\dot{Q}_T]\,[C_{\bar{v}}O_2])$

4. Equation 3 rewritten as the Fick equation:
   $VO_2 = [\dot{Q}_T]\,[C_aO_2 - C_{\bar{v}}O_2]$

5. Equation 4 rewritten as a function of cardiac output:
   $$\dot{Q}_T = \frac{VO_2}{([C_aO_2] - [C_{\bar{v}}O_2])\ (10)*}$$

* 10 is a constant that when multiplied by the a-v difference in the denominator of equation 5 converts the units of measure from milliliters of oxygen per deciliter of blood (ml/dL) into milliliters of oxygen per liter of blood (ml/liter).

One may divide the cardiac output into two components:

6. $\dot{Q}_T = \dot{Q}_C + \dot{Q}_S$

$\dot{Q}_C$ is the portion of the cardiac output (CO) that represents the function of the ideal lung: complete oxygenation of that blood volume. The $\dot{Q}_C$ is said to represent end-pulmonary capillary oxygen content (C_CO_2). The basis of this statement is that theoretically the oxygen level in this blood volume is at equilibrium with alveolar oxygen tension. This assumption is valid when hemoglobin transit time through the pulmonary capillary bed is normal and the P_AO_2 is 100 mmHg. The end-pulmonary capillary oxygen content is determined by predicting the ideal alveolar oxygen tension using the *ideal alveolar gas equation*. Since the P_AO_2 is the same as the P_aO_2, the P_AO_2 may be used in the calculation of the end-pulmonary capillary oxygen content. For example, Shapiro states that the ideal P_AO_2 at sea level and room air is 101 mmHg, therefore the ideal end-pulmonary capillary P_aO_2 is 101 mmHg.

$\dot{Q}_S$ is that portion of the CO that does not exchange with alveolar air (shunt). Since the shunted blood is not oxygenated by the lung, the oxygen content of the shunted blood reaching the left heart is the same value as the mixed venous oxygen content which is measured from the pulmonary artery.

Using the assumption concerning cardiac output ($\dot{Q}_T = \dot{Q}_C + \dot{Q}_S$) and the assumption that end-pulmonary capillary oxygen content can be obtained using the ideal alveolar gas equation,

7. $P_AO_2 = [P_B - P_{H2O}]\, F_IO_2 - P_aCO_2\, [1.25]$

There are additional steps that can be identified to understand how the shunt equation is mathematically derived:

8. $VO_2 = \dot{Q}_C\, [C_CO_2 - C_{\bar{v}}O_2]$

9. Equations 4 and 8 equal VO_2, therefore:
$\dot{Q}_T\, [C_aO_2 - C_{\bar{v}}O_2] = \dot{Q}_C\, [C_CO_2 - C_{\bar{v}}O_2]$

10. Looking back at equation 6:
$\dot{Q}_C = [\dot{Q}_T - \dot{Q}_S]$

11. Substituting:
$\dot{Q}_T\, [C_aO_2 - C_{\bar{v}}O_2] = [\dot{Q}_T - \dot{Q}_S]\, [C_CO_2 - C_{\bar{v}}O_2]$

12. Therefore:
$\dot{Q}_TC_aO_2 - \dot{Q}_TC_{\bar{v}}O_2 =$
$\dot{Q}_TC_CO_2 - \dot{Q}_TC_{\bar{v}}O_2 - \dot{Q}_SC_CO_2 - \dot{Q}_SC_{\bar{v}}O_2$

13. Therefore:
$\dot{Q}_S\, [C_CO_2 - C_{\bar{v}}O_2] = \dot{Q}_T\, [C_CO_2 - C_aO_2]$

14. *Classic Shunt Equation*:
$$\frac{\dot{Q}_S}{\dot{Q}_T} = \frac{[C_CO_2 - C_aO_2]}{[C_CO_2 - C_{\bar{v}}O_2]}$$

15. *Physiologic Shunt Equation*:
$$\frac{\dot{Q}_{sp}}{\dot{Q}_T} = \frac{[C_CO_2 - C_aO_2]}{[C_CO_2 - C_{\bar{v}}O_2]}$$

16. *Clinical Shunt Equation:*
$$\frac{\dot{Q}_{sp}}{\dot{Q}_T} = \frac{[C_CO_2 - C_aO_2]}{[C_aO_2 - C_{\bar{v}}O_2] + [C_CO_2 - C_aO_2]}$$

The physiologic shunt equation is another way of expressing equation 14, and they frequently are used interchangeably. However, there are some important differences. The $\dot{Q}_S$ in equation 14 is equivalent to true shunting, which is anatomic plus capillary shunting. The $\dot{Q}_{sp}$ in equation 15 includes true shunting plus some degree of venous admixture. Remember: Since $\dot{Q}_{sp}/\dot{Q}_T$ must be measured with the patient breathing less than 100% oxygen, there is an element of venous admixture contributing to the intrapulmonary shunt value. Also, the $\dot{Q}_{sp}/\dot{Q}_T$ does not require the measurement of the cardiac output.

You will notice that the clinical shunt equation incorporates arterial-venous oxygen content difference into the denominator in addition to the end-pulmonary capillary-mixed venous oxygen content difference. Shapiro explains that this addition makes it more apparent to the clinician that the cardiac output and oxygen consumption are important variables that affect the patient's shunt measurement. Therefore, the clinical shunt equation may be easier to understand and hence more directly applicable to the health care practitioner.

Additionally, Shapiro provides a detailed discussion of oxygen content terms accompanied by a pictorial representation of these terms as they relate to the physiologic shunt equation. This allows the reader to visualize oxygen content levels and how they change under various conditions. He describes how an acute pneumonitis affects mixed venous, arterial and end-capillary oxygen content and how an increase in the patient's cardiac output and F_IO_2 both singly and together will affect the patient's physiologic shunt.

When performing an intrapulmonary shunt measurement, one must have access to the patient's mixed venous oxygen content by means of a pulmonary artery catheter and arterial content by obtaining an arterial blood sample. The classic shunt equation is calculated when the patient is on an F_IO_2 of 1.0. This practice is no longer followed due to time limitations and also because many patients develop denitrogenation atelectasis and require higher maintenance F_IO_2 after being given 100% oxygen. It is recommended that the $\dot{Q}_{sp}/\dot{Q}_T$ be measured at the patient's maintenance F_IO_2. The patient's body position should also be noted when the $\dot{Q}_{sp}/\dot{Q}_T$ is measured. An important consideration when evaluating the results of a patient's shunt is his/her body position relative to the underlying lung pathology. If the diseased part of the lung is gravity-dependent, then the shunt will be higher than when the diseased lung is nongravity-dependent. If one is trying to assess improvement or deterioration in lung function, the body position must be consistent.

Prior to obtaining the arterial blood samples, the patient is kept undisturbed for 5 minutes. The arterial and pulmonary artery samples are drawn simultaneously, and hemodynamic values are measured close in time to the blood sampling.

There are specific rules followed for calculation of the C_aO_2, $C_{\bar{v}}O_2$ and C_CO_2:

- There should be 1 gm/dL difference between the C_aO_2 and $C_{\bar{v}}O_2$ hemoglobin content. If the difference is greater than 0.5 gm/dL hemoglobin, use the arithmetic average.
- Carbohemoglobin should be measured. If not, assume the level is 1.5%.

- Assume the P_{CO_2} is equal to the P_{AO_2}. If the P_{AO_2} is > 150 mmHg, the hemoglobin is 100% saturated.

- If the $P_{AO_2} > 125$ mmHg and < 150 mmHg: $C_{CO_2} = Hb\{(1.0 - HbCO) - 0.01\}\ \{1.34 + 0.0031\ (P_{AO_2})\}$

- If the $P_{AO_2} > 100$ mmHg and < 125 mmHg: $C_{CO_2} = Hb\{(1.0 - HbCO) - 0.02\}\ \{1.34 + 0.0031\ (P_{AO_2})\}$

If the patient does not require a pulmonary artery catheter, there are alternative methods that are used to reflect the patient's shunt. One can use these alternatives only if the patient has good cardiovascular function and a stable metabolic rate. Shapiro stresses that these alternative techniques require of the respiratory care practitioner a thorough understanding of the techniques' limitations so that the results are not overinterpreted.

Shapiro is a proponent of the estimated shunt equation technique for reflecting changes in the patient's physiologic shunt: $\dot{Q}_{sp}/\dot{Q}_T = C_{CO_2} - C_aO_2/3.5 + C_{CO_2} - C_aO_2$. The value 3.5 represents the $[C_{(a-v)}O_2]$ in the critically ill patient who has stable cardiovascular function. In order to determine the $C_{CO_2} - C_aO_2$, one must use the ideal gas equation. Remember that the ideal pulmonary end-capillary oxygen tension is considered to be equivalent to the alveolar oxygen tension. The product of the alveolar air equation is used in the calculation of C_{CO_2}. The patient's hemoglobin is 100% saturated and the P_{AO_2} (P_{CO_2}) is used to calculate the amount of oxygen dissolved in the plasma.

In addition to using the alveolar to arterial oxygen tension gradient in calculating the estimated shunt, the $P_{(A-a)}O_2$ is an alternative technique reflecting the patient's shunt. It is accurate and reliable when the patient's cardiovascular reserve and $C_{(a-v)}O_2$ are adequate and the P_aO_2 is > 150 mmHg. These qualifying factors limit its usefulness in the critically ill.

When the reliability of gas exchange indices are compared, the estimated shunt equation is the most reliable ($r = +0.94$). The other gas exchange indices lag behind. The respiratory index, a-A ratio and P/F ratio are more reliable assessment tools than the $P_{(A-a)}O_2$. The conclusion that must be drawn from these reliability results is that the estimated shunt equation is superior as an alternative shunt assessment tool to other oxygenation indices.

Key Points

- ➢ The shunt fraction is the best available means to identify the extent that the patient's hypoxemia is caused by pulmonary abnormalities.
- ➢ Intrapulmonary shunt is that portion of the patient's cardiac output that is not participating in gas exchange.
- ➢ The intrapulmonary shunt is subdivided into three components: anatomic shunt, capillary shunt and venous admixture.
- ➢ Normally, 2-5% of an individual's cardiac output bypasses the lung and enters directly into the left side of the heart. This is classified as an anatomic shunt.
- ➢ Atelectasis and consolidated pneumonia are examples of causes of a capillary shunt. The lung is not ventilated, but it is perfused by capillary blood.
- ➢ The sum of anatomic and capillary shunt is the true shunt. True shunt has a zero $\dot{V}/\dot{Q}$.
- ➢ Shunt effect is not a true shunt. It also reflects the contribution of low $\dot{V}/\dot{Q}$ to the patient's hypoxemia.
- ➢ When one measures the physiologic shunt, it includes the patient's true shunt and low $\dot{V}/\dot{Q}$ areas.
- ➢ *Physiologic shunt* and *venous admixture* are synonymous terms.
- ➢ Physiologic shunt is a more clinically relevant determination because it measures the patient's oxygenation impairment on his/her maintenance F_IO_2.
- ➢ The physiologic shunt is a derived value and does not require an absolute measure of the patient's cardiac output.
- ➢ The physiologic shunt can be measured only when both arterial and pulmonary artery blood samples are available.
- ➢ The classic shunt measure is determined when the patient is receiving 100% oxygen. The physiologic shunt measure is determined when the patient is on < 100% oxygen (maintenance F_IO_2).
- ➢ The body position should be noted when determining the physiologic shunt. If body position is not identified, one may make clinical judgements based on shunt measures that are not obtained using consistent methodology.
- ➢ When a shunt study is performed, the arterial and mixed venous blood samples should be drawn simultaneously and the hemodynamic measures should be obtained as close in time to the blood sampling as possible.
- ➢ The estimated shunt equation is a reliable alternative to the physiologic shunt in patients who have stable cardiovascular function and a stable metabolic rate.
- ➢ The estimated shunt equation is a reflection of the patient's shunt.

Formulas

Alveolar-arterial Oxygen Gradient

$P_{AO_2} - P_aO_2$

Alveolar Oxygen Ratio

$$\frac{P_aO_2}{P_AO_2}$$

Classic Shunt Equation

$$\frac{\dot{Q}_S}{\dot{Q}_T} = \frac{[C_CO_2 - C_aO_2]}{[C_CO_2 - C_{\bar{v}}O_2]}$$

Clinical Shunt Equation

$$\frac{\dot{Q}_{sp}}{\dot{Q}_T} = \frac{[C_CO_2 - C_aO_2]}{[C_aO_2 - C_{\bar{v}}O_2] + [C_CO_2 - C_aO_2]}$$

Estimated Shunt Equation

$$\frac{\dot{Q}_{sp}}{\dot{Q}_T} = \frac{[C_CO_2 - C_aO_2]}{3.5 + [C_CO_2 - C_aO_2]}$$

Fick Equation (Oxygen Consumption)

$$VO_2 = [\dot{Q}_T]\,([C_aO_2 - C_{\bar{v}}O_2])\,(10)$$

Fick Equation (Cardiac Output)

$$\frac{VO_2}{(\,[C_aO_2] - [C_{\bar{v}}O_2]\,)\,(10)}$$

Ideal Alveolar Gas Equation

$$P_AO_2 = [P_B - P_{H2O}]\,F_IO_2 - P_aCO_2\,[1.25]\,*$$

* For ease of calculation, the 0.8 has been converted to its reciprocal 1.25, allowing multiplication.

Oxygen Content

$$S_aO_2(Hb \times 1.34) + (PO_2 \times 0.0031)$$

Oxygenation ratio (P/F ratio)

$$\frac{P_aO_2}{F_IO_2}$$

Physiologic Shunt Equation

$$\frac{\dot{Q}_S}{\dot{Q}_T} = \frac{[C_CO_2 - C_aO_2]}{[C_CO_2 - C_{\bar{v}}O_2]}$$

Respiratory Index (RI)

$$\frac{P_{(A-a)}O_2}{P_aO_2}$$

Tables and Figures

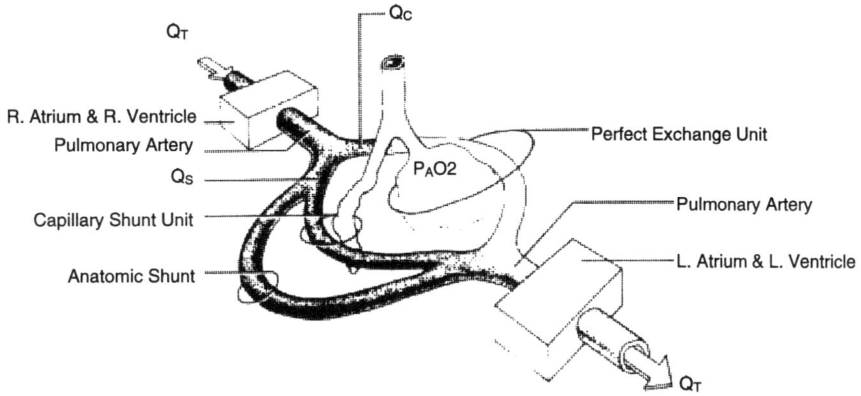

Figure 1: Mathematical concept of physiologic shunting (see text). $\dot{Q}_T$ is cardiac output per unit time; $\dot{Q}_C$ is the portion of the cardiac output that exchanges perfectly with alveolar air; $\dot{Q}_S$ is the portion of the cardiac output that does not exchange with alveolar air; P_AO_2 is the alveolar oxygen tension.

P_AO_2 = 101 mmHg
P_aO_2 = 95 mgHg
$P_{\bar{v}}O_2$ = 40 mmHg

Hgb = 15 gms
F_IO_2 = 0.21
Q_T = 5L
$C_{(a-v)}DO_2$ = 5 vol %
Q_{sp}/Q_T = 5%

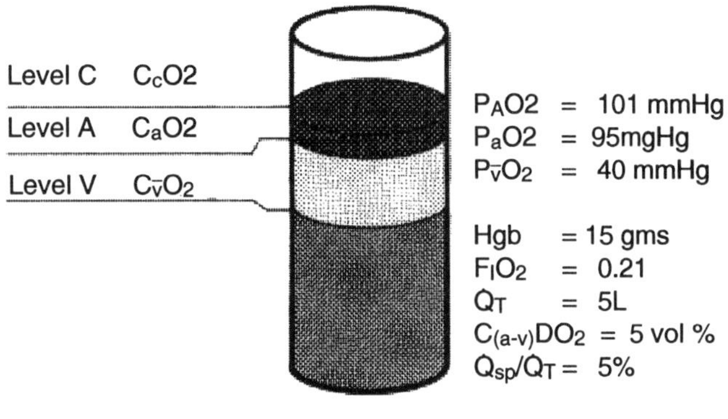

Figure 2: Schematic representation of the blood oxygen content levels in a normal individual. Representative normal values are listed for the major factors commonly affected in pathologic states. Level C: end-pulmonary capillary blood oxygen content level (C_cO_2). Level A: systemic arterial blood oxygen content level (C_aO_2). Level V: pulmonary arterial blood oxygen content level ($C_{\bar{v}}O_2$); P_AO_2, alveolar oxygen tension; P_aO_2, systemic arterial oxygen tension; $P_{\bar{v}}O_2$, pulmonary arterial oxygen tension; Hgb, hemoglobin content; F_IO_2, inspired oxygen fraction; Q_T, total cardiac output; $C_{(a-v)}DO_2$, arterial venous oxygen content difference [$C_{(a-v)}O_2$]; Q_{sp}/Q_T, calculated physiologic shunt.

$$\frac{Q_{sp}}{Q_T} = \frac{C_cO_2 - C_aO_2}{C_cO_2 - C_{\bar{v}}O_2} = \frac{\text{DIFF N}}{\text{DIFF D}}$$

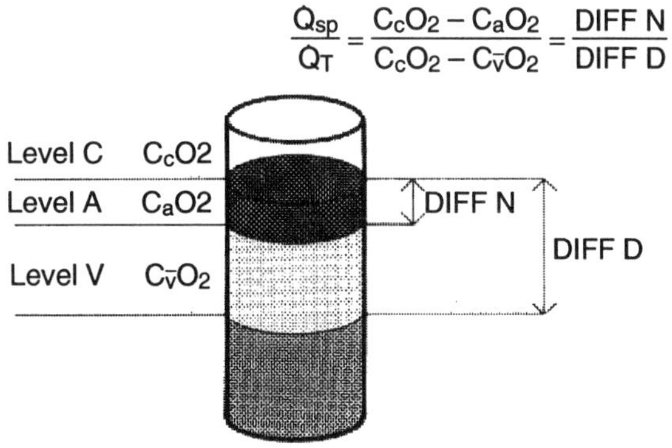

Figure 3: Oxygen content levels as they relate to the physiologic shunt equation. Q_{sp} = physiologic shunt, Q_T = total cardiac output, C_cO_2 = ideal end-pulmonary capillary oxygen content, C_aO_2 = systemic arterial oxygen content, $C_{\bar{v}}O_2$ = pulmonary arterial oxygen content. The numerator of the physiologic shunt equation (see text) is represented as Diff N (difference in the numerator); the denominator of the shunt equation is represented as Diff D (difference in the denominator). Changes of unequal magnitude between Diff N and Diff D will result in variations in the calculated physiologic shunt.

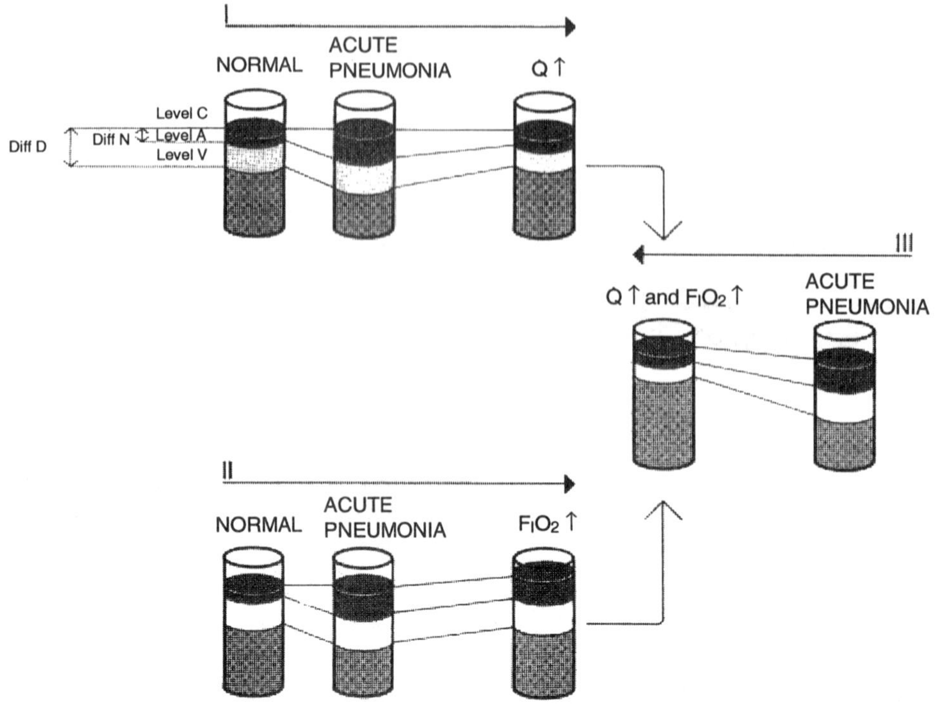

Figure 4: Schematic representation of changes in blood oxygen levels under various conditions. The purpose of this illustration is to conceptualize the difference between physiologic shunting and the hypoxemic effect of physiologic shunting. *I*, *II*, and *III* illustrate changes in a normal individual who contracts pneumonitis that causes a significant increase in intrapulmonary shunting without any compensatory physiologic change. The status from normal to *acute pneumonia* shows: no change in *Level C* because ventilation and F_IO_2 are unchanged, a significant drop in *Level A* due to increased shunting created by the pneumonia, and a drop in *Level V* because the AV content difference is unchanged (cardiac output and oxygen consumption unchanged). Since *DIFF N* has increased to a greater degree than *DIFF D*, the calculated shunt increases (see Fig. 7-4 in Clinical Application of Blood Gases). *Condition I* shows an increased cardiac output (Q ↑) in response to the acute hypoxemia. *Level C* remains unchanged sinnce neither ventilation nor F_IO_2 has been altered. The AV content difference has narrowed because the cardiac output has increased, while oxygen consumption remains unchanged. The increase in *Level V* results in a new dynamic equilibrium in which *Level A* is also increased. Note that the relatioship between *DIFF N* and *DIFF D* is only slightly altered. Thus, *Level A* (and therefore the P_aO_2) has increased with little change in the calculated shunt. In this instance the compensation for hypoxemia is cardiovascular; the intrapulmonary shunt has not changed. *Condition II* shows an increased inspired oxygen concentration (F_IO_2 ↑). *Level C* increases, while AV content difference remains unchanged (cardiac output and oxygen consumption unchanged). A new dynamic equilibrium results in *Level A* (and therefore the P_aO_2 increasing). The relationship between *DIFF N* and *DIFF D* is only slightly altered. *Level A* (and therefore P_aO_2) has increased with little change in the calculated shunt. In this instance, compensation for hypoxemia is via oxygen therapy; the intrapulmonary shunt is essentially unchanged. *Condition III* shows both cardiac output and inspired oxygen concentration changes (Q ↑ and F_IO_2 ↑). Note the profound increase in *Level A* (and therefore P_aO_2) with little alteration in the *DIFF N/DIFF D*.

Parameter	(Mean ± SD)		Range Min - Max	R Value
$\dot{Q}_{sp}/\dot{Q}_T$	22.3	(11.2)	3.0 - 53.0	
Estimated Shunt	27.6	(11.3)	2.7 - 62.3	+0.94
RI	3.1	(2.6)	0.3 - 14.0	+0.74
P_aO_2/P_AO_2	0.3	(0.2)	0.06 - 0.77	−0.72
P_aO_2/F_IO_2	1.8	(0.9)	0.1 - 4.3	−0.71
$P_{(A-a)}O_2$	222.8	(141.7)	32 - 611	+0.62

Table 1: Comparison of gas exchange indices.

Problems

Select and mark the best answer.

1. Which of the following is a definition of the term *intrapulmonary shunt*?
   a. The portion of the patient's ventilation that does not participate in gas exchange
   b. The portion of cardiac output that does not reach the tissues
   c. The portion of the cardiac output entering the left side of the heart that is not perfectly oxygenated by ideally ventilated alveoli
   d. The portion of the patient's alveolar ventilation that is perfused by the bronchial, pleural and thebesian veins

2. Perfusion in excess of ventilation is an example of what type of intrapulmonary shunt?
   a. Anatomic shunt
   b. Capillary shunt
   c. Venous admixture
   d. Estimated shunt

3. What is the portion of blood that enters the left side of the heart without traversing the pulmonary capillaries?
   a. Anatomic shunt
   b. Capillary shunt
   c. Venous admixture
   d. Estimated shunt

4. What is the portion of the cardiac output that traverses the pulmonary capillaries but does not participate in gas exchange with alveoli?
   a. Anatomic shunt
   b. Capillary shunt
   c. Venous admixture
   d. Estimated shunt

5. Which of the following is a description of zero shunt or true shunt?
   a. Shunt effect
   b. Estimated shunt
   c. Venous admixture
   d. The sum of anatomic and capillary shunts

6. In a normal person breathing room air, what type of shunt is the true measure of the individual's normal intrapulmonary shunt?
   a. Venous admixture
   b. Capillary shunt
   c. Physiologic shunt
   d. Estimated shunt

7. Using the Fick equation, which of the following physiologic variables is necessary for calculating cardiac output? (More than one answer may be correct.)
   a. Arteriovenous oxygen content difference
   b. End-pulmonary capillary oxygen content
   c. Oxygen consumption
   d. Physiologic shunt

8. The ideal alveolar PO_2 at sea level is ______________ .

9. Write the following equations:
   a. Fick equation

   b. Clinical shunt equation

c. Physiologic shunt equation

d. Estimated shunt equation

10. What is the difference between the classic shunt equation and the physiologic shunt equation?

____

____

____

____

11. Why should you keep the patient's body position the same when performing serial intrapulmonary shunt measurements?

____

____

____

____

12. If a patient with pneumonia has an increased cardiac output, how does an increase in blood flow modify the effects the pneumonia is having on the following physiologic variables?
Key: 1= increased, 2 = no change, 3 = decreased

_____ a. C_CO_2
_____ b. C_aO_2
_____ c. $C_{\bar{v}}O_2$
_____ d. a-v difference
_____ e. $\dot{Q}_{sp}/\dot{Q}_T$

13. Which of the following statements describes the difference between the physiologic shunt equation and the clinical shunt equation?
a. The clinical shunt equation is applied when the patient is on room air, while the physiologic shunt measurement is calculated when the patient is on 100% inspired oxygen.
b. The clinical shunt equation incorporates arterial-venous oxygen content difference in the denominator, while the physiologic shunt equation does not.
c. The clinical shunt equation is used to measure shunt in those patients who do not have a pulmonary artery catheter in place, while the physiologic shunt equation is used in those patients who are catheterized.
d. The clinical shunt equation can be used only in patients with stable cardiovascular systems and normal metabolic rates, while the physiologic shunt equation can be used in all situations.

14. If a patient with pneumonia is receiving supplemental oxygen, how will the increased F_IO_2 modify the effects the pneumonia is having on the following physiologic variables?
Key: 1 = increased, 2 = no change, 3 = decreased

_____ a. C_CO_2
_____ b. C_aO_2
_____ c. $C_{\bar{v}}O_2$
_____ d. a-v difference
_____ e. $\dot{Q}_{sp}/\dot{Q}_T$

15. When obtaining blood samples for intrapulmonary shunt measurement, what precautionary steps are recommended to ensure that the results will be valid and reliable?
a. If possible, the arterial and mixed venous blood samples should be drawn simultaneously.
b. The patient should not be stimulated for 30 minutes prior to sampling.
c. The patient's hemodynamic values should be obtained as close to the blood sampling time as possible.
d. Both a and c are correct.
e. a, b and c are correct.

16. If a patient with pneumonia is on supplemental oxygen and has an increase in cardiac output, how will the increased F_IO_2 and blood flow modify the effects the pneumonia is having on the following physiologic variables?
Key: 1 = increased, 2 = no change, 3 = decreased

_____ a. C_CO_2
_____ b. C_aO_2
_____ c. $C_{\bar{v}}O_2$
_____ d. a-v difference
_____ e. $\dot{Q}_{sp}/\dot{Q}_T$

17. When calculating the patient's intrapulmonary shunt, which of the following physiologic variables are obtained from the blood sample? (Place a check next to all correct answers.)

_____ a. C_CO_2
_____ b. C_aO_2
_____ c. Hemoglobin

_____ d. S_aO_2
_____ e. $C_{\bar{v}}O_2$
_____ f. $S_{\bar{v}}O_2$

18. Which alternative to shunt measurement is the most reliable reflection of physiologic shunt?
    a. $P_{(A-a)}O_2$
    b. P_aO_2/P_AO_2
    c. P_aO_2/F_IO_2
    d. Estimated shunt
    e. RI (respiratory index)

19. Which one of the following oxygen tension indices has the highest correlation to the physiologic shunt?
    a. $P_{(A-a)}O_2$
    b. P_aO_2/P_AO_2
    c. P_aO_2/F_IO_2
    d. RI (respiratory index)
    e. Dissolved oxygen content

20. Under what clinical conditions may the $P_{(A-a)}O_2$ be used to reflect intrapulmonary shunting? (More than one answer may be correct.)
    a. The patient must have adequate cardiopulmonary reserve and an adequate arterial-venous oxygen content difference.
    b. The patient must have an arterial oxygen tension above 150 mmHg.
    c. The patient must be receiving 100% inspired oxygen concentration.
    d. The patient must have an intrapulmonary shunt ≤ 30%.

21. A 26-year-old man was admitted with severe pneumonia. Initially, he was placed on a nasal cannula at 3 L/min. He worsened throughout the evening and eventually was intubated and mechanically ventilated. A pulmonary artery catheter was placed after he was intubated. With the clinical data given, calculate the following:

    a. Estimated shunt:

Hb 14 gm%	BP 150/84	T 38.1° C
Hct 42%	HR 130 beats/min	RR 44 bpm

    P_B 735 mmHg, P_{H_2O} 49.4
    Blood gases: pH 7.38, PCO_2 45, PO_2 47, S_aO_2 82% on 40% venturi mask

    b. Physiologic shunt:

Hb 14 gm%	BP 114/76	T 38.1° C
Hct 42%	HR 130 beats/min	RR 20 bpm

    P_B 735 mmHg, P_{H_2O} 49.4
    Pulmonary artery values: PAP 34/19 mmHg
    PCWP 16 mmHg, RAP 12 mmHg, CO 5.16 LPM
    Blood gases on CMV: F_IO_2 0.5, PEEP 13
    Arterial pH 7.49, PCO_2 35, PO_2 65, S_aO_2 93%
    Mixed venous pH 7.47, PCO_2 38, PO_2 36, $S_{\bar{v}}O_2$ 68%

    c. Oxygen consumption:

Hb 14 gm%	BP 114/76	T 38.1° C
Hct 42%	HR 130 beats/min	RR 20 bpm

    P_B 735 mmHg, P_{H_2O} 49.4
    Pulmonary artery values: PAP 34/19 mmHg
    PCWP 16 mmHg, RAP 12 mmHg, CO 5.16 LPM
    Blood gases on CMV: F_IO_2 0.5, PEEP 13
    Arterial pH 7.49, PCO_2 35, PO_2 65, S_aO_2 93%
    Mixed venous pH 7.47, PCO_2 38, PO_2 36, $S_{\bar{v}}O_2$ 68%

Answers to Problems

1. c: The portion of the cardiac output entering the left side of the heart that is not perfectly oxygenated by ideally ventilated alveoli.

2. c: Low ventilation/perfusion is a problem that typically causes venous admixture. Venous admixture is often referred to as low $\dot{V}/\dot{Q}$, $\dot{V}/\dot{Q}$ inequity or shunt effect. An anatomic or capillary shunt would cause zero $\dot{V}/\dot{Q}$ or true shunt. The estimated shunt is an alternative method used to assess the patient's shunt when it is not possible to obtain a mixed venous blood sample.

3. a: Anatomic shunt is that portion of the cardiac output that bypasses the pulmonary capillaries. It anatomically is directed to the left side of the heart without being oxygenated by the lung. Every individual has a 2-5% anatomic shunt. Right-to-left intracardiac shunts and vascular tumors will increase the patient's anatomic shunt and may severely impair oxygenation.

4. b: Capillary shunt is that portion of the cardiac output that traverses the lungs but does not participate in gas exchange. This type of shunt is minimal in the individual with normal lungs. Lung disorders or diseases such as atelectasis and consolidated pneumonia will cause a capillary shunt. After the lung disease is treated or the condition is reversed, then the capillary shunt returns to zero or baseline.

5. d: Zero shunt or true shunt is the sum of the anatomic shunt and the capillary shunt. Shunt effect and venous admixture represent the oxygenation impairment due to low $\dot{V}/\dot{Q}$ units. The estimated shunt is an alternative measure that can be used to reflect the physiologic shunt.

6. c: When measuring intrapulmonary shunt, the physiologic shunt is measured at less than 100% inspired oxygen. Therefore, this measure is the best tool to ascertain the shunt of the individual who is breathing 21% oxygen.

7. a, c: $CO = \frac{VO_2}{([C_aO_2] - [C_{\bar{v}}O_2])\ (10)}$

Arteriovenous oxygen content difference and oxygen consumption are both necessary for calculation of cardiac output using the Fick equation. The end-pulmonary capillary oxygen content is used in shunt calculation. The physiologic shunt determines the percentage of the cardiac output that does not participate in gas exchange. The equation does not identify the entire cardiac output.

8. 101 mmHg: The ideal alveolar PO_2 at room air and at sea level is considered to be 101 mmHg. If all of the cardiac output exchanges perfectly with perfectly ventilated alveoli, then the P_AO_2 would be equal to the P_aO_2. In this situation, there is no intrapulmonary shunt.

9. Fick Equation (Oxygen Consumption):

$$VO_2 = [\dot{Q}_T]\ ([C_aO_2 - C_{\bar{v}}O_2])\ (10)$$

Clinical Shunt Equation:

$$\frac{\dot{Q}_{sp}}{\dot{Q}_T} = \frac{[C_cO_2 - C_aO_2]}{[C_aO_2 - C_{\bar{v}}O_2] + [C_cO_2 - C_aO_2]}$$

Physiologic Shunt Equation:

$$\frac{\dot{Q}_{sp}}{\dot{Q}_T} = \frac{[C_cO_2 - C_aO_2]}{[C_cO_2 - C_{\bar{v}}O_2]}$$

Estimated Shunt Equation:

$$\frac{\dot{Q}_{sp}}{\dot{Q}_T} = \frac{[C_cO_2 - C_aO_2]}{3.5 + [C_cO_2 - C_aO_2]}$$

10. The classic shunt equation concept assumes that the patient is receiving 100% oxygen. This equation measures the true shunt or zero $\dot{V}/\dot{Q}$ but not venous admixture. The physiologic shunt equation measures the intrapulmonary shunt on individuals receiving less than 100% oxygen. This value includes anatomic and capillary shunt as well as venous admixture at the patient's maintenance F_IO_2. This value is a better reflection of the lung's oxygenation performance.

11. Shunt can be measured in any body position. However, because the distribution of pulmonary perfusion changes with body position, it is important to keep the patient's position the same for all shunt determinations in order to maintain intersample consistency. If body position is the not the same in all shunt determinations, the fluctuations in shunt may be caused by either position changes or actual improvement or worsening of lung function.

12. a. 2: Increased cardiac output will have no effect on the patient's C_cO_2 because there is no change in ventilation and F_IO_2.

    b. 1: The C_aO_2 increases secondary to the improvement in cardiovascular function. The increase in venous content with no change in metabolic rate results in an increase in the arterial content.

    c. 1: The $C_{\bar{v}}O_2$ increases secondary to the increased blood flow to the tissue without an increase in the metabolic rate. This results in a net increase in venous oxygen content. The increase in $C_{\bar{v}}O_2$ changes homeostasis and increases the C_aO_2.

    d. 3: Arteriovenous content difference is decreased because cardiac output has increased while the oxygen consumption remains unchanged.

    e. 2: Because of the cardiovascular compensation, the oxygen and venous content increased but the underlying pulmonary problem is still present. Therefore, the physiologic shunt is relatively unchanged.

13. b: The appearance of arterial-venous content difference in the denominator of the equation makes the concept of cardiac output and metabolic rate more prominent in the equation. It is suggested that when all the physiologic variables are prominent, the concept of shunt is clear and understandable.

14. a. 1: Increased F_IO_2 will increase the patient's C_cO_2 because there was a change in F_IO_2 which increases the P_AO_2.

    b. 1: The C_aO_2 increases secondary to the improved oxygenation in low $\dot{V}/\dot{Q}$ lung units. This reduces the contribution of venous admixture to the patient's hypoxemia.

    c. 1: The $C_{\bar{v}}O_2$ increases secondary to the increased C_aO_2.

    d. 2: Arteriovenous content difference is not changed because cardiac output and oxygen consumption are unchanged.

    e. 2: Because of the compensation secondary to the increase in F_IO_2, the P_aO_2 and C_aO_2 increased but the physiologic shunt remained unchanged. The underlying cause of the pulmonary problem is still present.

15. d: The patient should remain undisturbed for 5 minutes prior to blood sampling. Arterial and venous blood samples should be drawn simultaneously, if possible. Finally, the hemodynamic values should be measured as close to the sampling time as possible.

16. a. 1: Increased F_IO_2 will increase the patient's C_CO_2 because there was a change in F_IO_2 which increases the P_AO_2.

    b. 1: The C_aO_2 increases secondary to the improved oxygenation in low $\dot{V}/\dot{Q}$ lung units and improvement in cardiovascular function.

    c. 1: The $C_{\bar{v}}O_2$ increases secondary to the increased C_aO_2 and cardiac output.

    d. 3: Arteriovenous content difference is decreased because cardiac output has increased while the oxygen consumption remains unchanged. Despite the increase in the C_aO_2, the $C_{\bar{v}}O_2$ increases more dramatically and narrows the a-v difference.

    e. 2: Because of the compensation secondary to the increase in F_IO_2 and cardiovascular function, the C_aO_2 increased but the physiologic shunt remained unchanged. The underlying cause of the pulmonary problem is still present.

17. b: The C_aO_2 is obtained by using the P_aO_2 and S_aO_2 from the arterial blood gas. The hemoglobin reading is obtained from the patient's current hemoglobin.

    c: The hemoglobin is used in the calculation of arterial and venous oxygen content. It must be drawn from the patient's blood. It is not an assumed value.

    d: The S_aO_2 is determined from the patient's arterial blood gas. It will fluctuate with the P_aO_2.

    e: The $C_{\bar{v}}O_2$ is obtained by using the $P_{\bar{v}}O_2$ and $S_{\bar{v}}O_2$ from the mixed venous blood gas obtained through the pulmonary artery catheter. The hemoglobin reading is obtained from a venous blood sample.

    f: The $S_{\bar{v}}O_2$ is determined from the patient's mixed venous blood gas. It will fluctuate with the $P_{\bar{v}}O_2$.

18. d: The estimated shunt equation correlates the most closely with the physiologic shunt equation.

19. d: The respiratory index (RI) is a good alternative method to reflect the patient's shunt. The estimated shunt equation is the most reliable alternative. But if patient circumstances prohibit the use of the estimated shunt equation, the RI is a reasonable assessment tool.

20. a, b: The $P_{(A\text{-}a)}O_2$ is a useful tool to reflect intrapulmonary shunting when the patient has adequate cardiopulmonary reserve and adequate a-v oxygen content difference. The P_aO_2 must also reflect 100% Hb saturation ($P_aO_2 > 150$ mmHg).

21. a. 53%:

Estimated Shunt Equation

$$\frac{\dot{Q}_{SP}}{\dot{Q}_T} = \frac{[C_CO_2 - C_aO_2]}{3.5 + [C_CO_2 - C_aO_2]}$$

$$C_CO_2 = 1.00\,(14 \times 1.34) + (218 \text{ mmHg} \times 0.0031)$$
$$19.44 \text{ ml/dL} = 18.76 \text{ ml/dL} + .676 \text{ ml/dL}$$

$$C_aO_2 = .82(14 \times 1.34) + (47 \text{ mmHg} \times 0.0031)$$
$$15.53 \text{ ml/dL} = 15.38 \text{ ml/dL} + .146 \text{ ml/dL}$$

With the above information, the $\dot{Q}_{sp}/\dot{Q}_T$ can now be calculated:

$$\frac{\dot{Q}_{SP}}{\dot{Q}_T} = \frac{19.44 \text{ ml/dL} - 15.53 \text{ ml/dL}}{3.5 + [19.44 \text{ ml/dL} - 15.53 \text{ ml/dL}]}$$

$$= \frac{3.91 \text{ ml/dL}}{3.5 \text{ ml/dL} + 3.91 \text{ ml/dL}}$$

$$= \frac{3.91 \text{ ml/dL}}{7.41 \text{ ml/dL}} \times 100$$

$$\frac{\dot{Q}_{SP}}{\dot{Q}_T} = 53\%$$

b. 30%:

Physiologic Shunt Equation

$$\frac{\dot{Q}_{SP}}{\dot{Q}_T} = \frac{[C_CO_2 - C_aO_2]}{[C_CO_2 - C_{\bar{v}}O_2]}$$

$$C_CO_2 = 1.00\,(14 \times 1.34) + (299 \text{ mmHg} \times 0.0031)$$
$$19.69 \text{ ml/dL} = 18.76 \text{ ml/dL} + .927 \text{ ml/dL}$$

$$C_aO_2 = .93(14 \times 1.34) + (65 \text{ mmHg} \times 0.0031)$$
$$17.65 \text{ ml/dL} = 17.45 \text{ ml/dL} + .201 \text{ ml/dL}$$

$$C_{\bar{v}}O_2 = .68(14 \times 1.34) + (65 \text{ mmHg} \times 0.0031)$$
$$12.87 \text{ ml/dL} = 12.76 \text{ ml/dL} + .112 \text{ ml/dL}$$

With the above information, the $\dot{Q}_{sp}/\dot{Q}_T$ can now be calculated:

$$\frac{\dot{Q}_{SP}}{\dot{Q}_T} = \frac{19.69 \text{ ml/dL} - 17.65 \text{ ml/dL}}{19.69 \text{ ml/dL} - 12.87 \text{ ml/dL}}$$

$$= \frac{2.04 \text{ ml/dL}}{6.82 \text{ ml/dL}}$$

$$= .2991 \times 100$$

$$\frac{\dot{Q}_{SP}}{\dot{Q}_T} = 30\%$$

c. 247 ml/min:

Fick Equation (Oxygen Consumption)

$VO_2 = [\dot{Q}_T]\ ([C_aO_2 - C_{\bar{v}}O_2])\ (10)$

$= 5.16\ L/min \times \{10\ dL/L\ (17.65\ ml/dL - 12.87\ ml/dL)\}$

$= 5.16\ L/min \times \{10\ dL/L\ (4.78\ ml/dL)\}$

$= 246.648\ ml/min$

Case Study

This 22-year-old white female was admitted for treatment of ARDS secondary to aspiration pneumonia. The patient aspirated a small amount of concentrated gastric juice prior to intubation for a caesarian section. She was treated at the local hospital with antibiotics and mechanical ventilation but was transferred to a tertiary care center when she developed bilateral pneumothoraces.

Physical Exam:
Oriented 22-year-old white female in no apparent distress.

Nasotracheal tube in the right naris, bilateral chest tubes in place.

Vital signs: P = 100
RR = 15
BP = 128/78, afebrile

Height 5'5", Weight 60 kg

Chest: Bilateral breath sounds including wheezes and crackles. Chest x-ray showed 5 lobe infiltrates and visible air bronchogram.
Impression: ARDS secondary to aspiration
Initial procedures performed: Left radial arterial line inserted, insertion of pulmonary artery catheter

Day 1: The patient is receiving mechanical ventilation with a V_T of 750 ml, RR 10, F_IO_2 1.0, PEEP 15 cm H_2O. Breath sounds were clear and decreased. Minimal secretions were suctioned from the nasotracheal tube. The F_IO_2 was decreased to 0.7.

Vital signs: BP = 140/85
HR = 120
T = 37.3° C

Lab studies: Hb 9.6 gm/dL, Hct 28%, WBC 26.6/mm^3, RBC 3.1 million/mm^3, Electrolytes WNL, Renal function normal

Blood gas results on CMV: F_IO_2 0.7, PEEP 15 cm H_2O, V_T 750 ml, RR 10
pH 7.43, P_aCO_2 37 mmHg, P_aO_2 85 mmHg, S_aO_2 96%
pH 7.40, $P_{\bar{v}}CO_2$ 43 mmHg, $P_{\bar{v}}O_2$ 33 mmHg, $S_{\bar{v}}O_2$ 62%

Hemodynamic values: Mean PAP 38 mmHg,
RA 11 mmHg, CO 4.0 L/min, SVR 1085 dynes sec cm^{-5}

Day 2: The PEEP was increased to 20 cm H_2O. The patient developed a GI bleed thought to be secondary to stress.

Vital signs: BP = 150/100
HR = 140
T = 37.1° C

Lab studies: Hb 10.6 gm/dL, Hct 31%, WBC 26.6 /mm^3, RBC 3.43 million/mm^3, Electrolytes WNL, Renal function normal

Blood gas results on CMV: F_IO_2 0.7, PEEP 20 cm H_2O, V_T 750 ml, RR 10
pH 7.42, P_aCO_2 44 mmHg, P_aO_2 107 mmHg, S_aO_2 99%
pH 7.39, $P_{\bar{v}}CO_2$ 48 mmHg, $P_{\bar{v}}O_2$ 28 mmHg, $S_{\bar{v}}O_2$ 52%

Hemodynamic values: Mean PAP 38 mmHg,
PCWP 15 mmHg, CO 1.9 L/min, SVR 1882 dynes sec cm^{-5}

1. Would you use the estimated shunt equation in this patient situation? Explain your answer.

2. Using the data provided on Day 1, calculate the following (use a barometric pressure of 740 mmHg):
   a. Alveolar-arterial oxygen gradient
   b. Oxygenation ratio
   c. Oxygen tension to inspired oxygen concentration ratio
   d. Respiratory index
   e. Physiologic shunt

3. Looking at the results of question 2, are the above values consistent within themselves? Explain your answer.

4. Looking at the information provided in the patient's second hospital day, how would you assess the patient's response to the increase in PEEP? Is the patient tolerating the change in therapy?

5. Using the knowledge you gained in Chapters 4 and 7, determine what patient problems would affect her oxygen carrying capacity and oxygen delivery to the tissues.

6. Using the Fick equation, calculate the patient's oxygen consumption on Day 2. Discuss the results.

7. Discuss what the physiologic significance of a $P_{\bar{v}}O_2$ of 33 mmHg represents.

8. Looking at Day 2, discuss this patient's cardiopulmonary reserve. Is it adequate? Is it efficient?

Suggested Additional Readings

Kacmarek, RM, Mack, CW and Dimas, S, *The Essentials of Respiratory Care,* 3rd edition, C.V. Mosby, St. Louis, MO, 1990, pp. 179-188, 198-199.

Scanlan, CL, Spearman, CB and Sheldon, RL, *Egan's Fundamentals of Respiratory Care,* 5th edition, C.V. Mosby, St. Louis, MO, 1990, pp. 205-206, 209-214, 333-335, 340-344.

Shapiro, BA, Kacmarek, RM, Cane, RD, Peruzzi, WT and Hauptman, D, *Clinical Application of Respiratory Care*, 4th edition, Mosby-Year Book, St. Louis, MO, 1991, Chapter 14.

CHAPTER 8

Assessment of Cellular Oxygenation

Objectives

After reading Chapter 8 and successfully completing this chapter of the workbook the student will be able to:

1. Define the following terms:

antioxidant mechanism	oxygen carrying capacity
$C\bar{v}O_2$	oxygen consumption
decompensation	oxygen delivery
derived value	oxygen demand (DO_2)
ectopy	oxygen extraction ration
extravascular fluid (EVF)	oxygen reservoir
hypercarbia	reducing substance
interpulmonary shunting	reference value
mixed venous oxygen status	shunted blood
oxidizing substance	$S\bar{v}O_2$

2. Given appropriate data, calculate the following values:
   a. $C_{(a-v)}O_2$
   b. $S\bar{v}O_2$
   c. DO_2
   d. OER
   e. O_2 Del
   f. VO_2
3. Differentiate between reducing and oxidizing substances.
4. Explain the effects of high oxygen levels on cell components.
5. Discuss the concept of optimum biological activity with respect to cellular oxygen tension.
6. Describe two processes which protect us from damage due to high cellular oxygen levels.
7. Describe what is meant by the term *mixed venous blood.*
8. Explain the reasons for and value of obtaining mixed venous blood samples.
9. State the appropriate sampling site from which a mixed venous sample should be obtained.
10. State the normal values of $P\bar{v}O_2$, $S\bar{v}O_2$, $P\bar{v}CO_2$, venous pH and $C_{(a-v)}O_2$.
11. State complications which can arise as a result of cardiac catheter misplacement.
12. Explain the two reasons why critically ill patients may have abnormal $C_{(a-v)}O_2$ values.
13. State the direction of change in $C_{(a-v)}O_2$ values for each reason stated in objective 12.
14. State the normal value and explain the concept of oxygen consumption.
15. State the normal value of oxygen extraction and the oxygen extraction ratio (OER).
16. Explain the derivation of the oxygen extraction value.
17. Demonstrate that $C_{(a-v)}O_2$ and VO_2 are not the same entity.
18. Explain the value of determining $C_{(a-v)}O_2$ when attempting to assess cardiac output ($\dot{Q}_T$) effectiveness.
19. List four factors which influence the accuracy of pulmonary artery (PA) blood gas samples.
20. State two reasons that it may be wrong to assume that oxygen consumption is stable in critically ill patients.
21. Describe a compensatory mechanism for hypoxemia secondary to interpulmonary shunting.
22. Discuss the clinical meaning of an increase in the oxygen extraction ratio.
23. State the formula for calculating $S\bar{v}O_2$.
24. Explain the concept of O_2 Del.
25. State the effects of different levels of P_aO_2 on O_2 Del.
26. Discuss the role of extravascular fluid (EVF) in maintaining cellular PO_2.
27. Describe the interaction of O_2 and hemoglobin in the "steep portion" of the oxyhemoglobin dissociation curve.

Definitions

antioxidant mechanism Protective activities which prevent or reduce the effects of high oxygen levels in the cells.

C_aO_2 Oxygen carrying capacity of arterial blood.

cardiac output ($\dot{Q}_T$) Volume of blood ejected by the heart per minute; it is a product of stroke volume multiplied by heart rate per minute.

$C\bar{v}O_2$ Oxygen carrying capacity of venous blood.

decompensation Changes in physiologic or biochemical processes which result in adverse changes in ("normal") diagnostic values.

dL decaliter; one tenth of a liter = 100 ml (1 liter = 1000 ml; 1000 ml/10 = 1 decaliter).

ectopy An event happening at the wrong time, e.g., a premature ventricular contraction.

extravascular fluid (EVF) Bodily fluids (normal or otherwise) which exist outside the vascular system bathing the tissues and cells.

hypercarbia Increased levels of carbon dioxide in a substance (hypercarboxemia: in the blood).

interpulmonary shunting Pulmonary capillary blood flow which does not take part in gas exchange. From an oxygenation and carbon dioxide excretion standpoint, this is wasted perfusion. A method of expressing ventilation-perfusion mismatch.

mixed venous blood A combination of shunted (high oxygen, low carbon dioxide) blood and true venous (low oxygen, high carbon dioxide) blood found in the pulmonary artery.

mixed venous oxygen status The oxygen saturation of mixed venous blood.

optimum biological activity The cellular oxygen tension at which the maximum energy is produced at the lowest level of cellular damage due to the toxic effects of high oxygen levels.

oxygen carrying capacity (C_aO_2 or $C_{\bar{v}}O_2$) The maximum amount of oxygen which can be carried in 100 ml of blood.

oxygen consumption (VO_2) The amount of oxygen removed from the blood and utilized in the cells for metabolic processes.

oxygen delivery (DO_2) The amount of oxygen delivered to the tissues (cells) by the arterial blood.

oxygen demand (DO_2) The amount of oxygen required by the cells to maintain adequate aerobic metabolic energy production.

oxygen extraction ($C_{(a\text{-}v)}O_2$) The amount of oxygen removed from 100 ml of systemic blood per minute. The arterial to mixed venous oxygen difference expressed in ml/dL.

oxygen extraction ratio (OER) The amount of oxygen extraction per arterial oxygen content ($C_{(a\text{-}v)}O_2/C_aO_2$).

oxygen reservoir The biological storage site of oxygen in higher order animals; the hemoglobin.

oxidizing agent A substance which adds hydrogen to a system by giving up oxygen, making the substance more acidic.

reducing agent A substance which removes hydrogen from a biochemical system, reducing the acidity of the system.

reference value A value which is actually measured or observed.

shunted blood Blood which bypasses a site of physiologic activity. In pulmonary medicine, blood which does not take part in gas exchange at either the cellular (tissue) or alveolar level.

$S_{\bar{v}}O_2$ Mixed venous oxygen saturation.

Introduction

In Chapter 8 Shapiro describes a method of determining the adequacy of cellular oxygenation.

The initial discussion summarizes the damaging effects of high (oxidizing) levels of oxygen on cell structures balanced with the increase in energy production in cells with elevated oxygen levels. Shapiro defines the optimum biological activity level as that level of oxygen tension at which the highest energy output is gained for the least amount of cellular damage. He states that the two most important antioxidant mechanisms in the body are biological barriers (tissue and fluids which separate the high oxygen concentrations for the cellular organelles) and the presence of high nitrogen levels (biologically inert gases) in the blood and alveoli.

Shapiro chooses the arterial to venous content difference ($C_{(a\text{-}v)}O_2$) as the most effective and efficient method of assessing cellular oxygenation. Shapiro points out that the difference between the arterial O_2 content and the venous O_2 content is oxygen which has diffused into the extracellular (extravascular) fluid. He then describes the oxygenation characteristics of the heart's ventricles (right ventricle — systemic venous drainage; left ventricle — pulmonary capillary drainage). He points out that placement of mixed venous sampling catheters is critically important if acceptable and accurate samples are to be obtained with a minimum of risk. The pulmonary artery is the safest and most accurate site from which to obtain samples for $C_{(a\text{-}v)}O_2$ determination according to Shapiro.

Normal volunteers have venous blood gas values within the following ranges: $P_{\bar{v}}O_2$ 40 mmHg, $P_{\bar{v}}CO_2$ 44-46 mmHg, pH 7.34-7.36. The normal value of $C_{(a\text{-}v)}O_2$ is 5 ml/dL. Critically ill patients will have one of two outcomes in terms of effects on $C_{(a\text{-}v)}O_2$. Those patients with adequate cardiopulmonary reserves who have cardiac outputs ($\dot{Q}_T$) which increase in excess of oxygen consumption will have decreased $C_{(a\text{-}v)}O_2$. Patients with decreased cardiopulmonary reserves will initially have an increased $C_{(a\text{-}v)}O_2$, then frank decompensation will occur. It is important to note that these changes usually occur prior to changes in arterial oxygen tension (P_aO_2).

Oxygen consumption (VO_2) is the amount of oxygen utilized by the body during aerobic metabolic processes in one minute (ml/min). It is determined by calculating the arterial to venous oxygen content difference times cardiac output times 10: $VO_2 = C_{(a-v)}O_2 \times \dot{Q}_T \times 10$.

Oxygen extraction ($C_{(a-v)}O_2$) is the amount of oxygen removed from the arterial systemic blood flow by the tissues in ml/dL (or vol%). This value is determined by calculating the difference between the oxygen content per 100 ml of arterial blood and that of 100 ml of venous blood. If the VO_2 is constant, $C_{(a-v)}O_2$ varies inversely with the cardiac output ($\dot{Q}_T$). Therefore, $C_{(a-v)}O_2$ provides an estimate of how well $\dot{Q}_T$ is responding to the body's metabolic oxygen requirements.

Mixed venous oxygen saturation ($S\bar{v}O_2$) is dependent on the amount of intrapulmonary shunting. $C_{(a-v)}O_2$ is inversely related to the $C\bar{v}O_2$ and the $S\bar{v}O_2$. Decreasing the $C_{(a-v)}O_2$ by increasing the cardiac output will increase the $C\bar{v}O_2$ and the $S\bar{v}O_2$.

Shapiro indicates that the oxygen extraction ratio (OER: $C_{(a-v)}O_2/C_aO_2$) reflects the oxygen taken up by the tissue. This is expressed as a percentage of the arterial oxygen content. Normally 25% of the arterial oxygen content is extracted by the tissues (C_aO_2 = 20 ml/dL; $C\bar{v}O_2$ = 15 ml/dL). Oxygen extraction ratios greater than 25% indicate either a reduced arterial oxygen content or inadequate cardiac output to meet the tissue oxygen requirements. Note: If P_aO_2 is greater than 60 mmHg (S_aO_2 > 90%), oxygen delivery (DO_2) is mainly dependent on Hb content and $\dot{Q}_T$.

Mixed venous oxygen status is the difference between the oxygen delivered to the tissues (DO_2) and the oxygen extracted by the tissues ($C_{(a-v)}O_2$). Shapiro maintains that when an adequate quantity of oxygen is available in the systemic capillaries (i.e., getting to the tissues), inadequate cellular oxygenation is not due to either heart or lung dysfunction. The normal value of DO_2 is 1000ml/min ($DO_2 = C_aO_2 \times \dot{Q}_T \times 10$). Remember that if the P_aO_2 is greater than 60 mmHg (S_aO_2 > 90%), oxygen delivery (DO_2) is dependent on the Hb content and $\dot{Q}_T$.

When P_aO_2 exceeds 100 mmHg, little additional benefit accrues to oxygen delivery because of the shape of the oxyhemoglobin dissociation curve. Ideally, PO_2 should equilibrate between capillary blood and extravascular fluid (EVF). EVF has 5-10 times the fluid volume of the systemic capillaries. P_aO_2s greater than 60 mmHg do little to improve venous capillary PO_2. Thus, a P_aO_2 higher than 60 mmHg will have little effect on oxygen extraction ($C_{(a-v)}O_2$).

Key Points

- High intracellular oxygen levels increase energy production.
- These same high intracellular oxygen levels cause damage to cell organelles.
- The intracellular oxygen tension level ($P_{ic}O_2$) which produces the most energy at the lowest level of damage is called the optimum biological activity level.
- Normal $P_{ic}O_2$ is 0.6 mmHg.
- Complex biological systems have antioxidative mechanisms to protect the cell from oxidative damage.
- The high percentage of nitrogen in the atmosphere and the body suppresses the oxidative effects of oxygen.
- The relatively large anatomical distances between high oxygen levels in the blood and the tissues serve to protect the cells from oxidative damage.
- Cellular (tissue) oxygenation must be assessed indirectly.
- We can indirectly reflect cellular oxygenation using available clinical information.
- The difference between arterial and venous oxygen content approximates the amount of oxygen that diffuses into extravascular fluid.
- Right ventricular (RV) blood is representative of systemic venous drainage (venous: deoxygenated blood).
- Left ventricular (LV) blood is derived from the pulmonary capillaries (arterial: oxygenated blood).
- $C_{(a-v)}O_2$ (arterial to venous oxygen difference) is calculated using data obtained by analyzing arterial oxygen content and the oxygen content of pulmonary artery (PA) blood (venous blood).
- The most reliable and consistent source of mixed venous oxygen content data is from pulmonary artery catheters.
- Catheters placed in the vena cava, right atrium and right ventricle are not useful due to grossly variable oxygen content.
- Normal mixed venous blood gas values are pH 7.34-7.36, $P\bar{v}CO_2$ 44-46 mmHg, $P\bar{v}O_2$ 40 mmHg.
- Normal $C_{(a-v)}O_2$ is 5 ml/dL.
- Due to increased oxygen consumption with reduced oxygen extraction, those critically ill patients with good cardiopulmonary reserves will increase cardiac output ($\dot{Q}_T$) and will exhibit a decrease in $C_{(a-v)}O_2$.
- Patients who cannot increase $\dot{Q}_T$ will exhibit increasing $C_{(a-v)}O_2$, eventually above the "normal" value.
- Changes in $C_{(a-v)}O_2$ often occur before significant changes in P_aO_2.
- Oxygen consumption (VO_2) is ($C_IO_2 - C_EO_2$)/minute.

- Normal VO_2 is 250 ml/minute.
- The amount of blood removed from 100 ml of arterial blood by the tissues is called the oxygen extraction.
- Normal resting oxygen extraction is 5 ml/dL (5 vol%); this is the $C_{(a-v)}O_2$.
- Oxygen extraction ($C_{(a-v)}O_2$) is not the same as oxygen consumption (VO_2).
- For any VO_2, $C_{(a-v)}O_2$ will vary inversely with the cardiac output ($\dot{Q}_T$).
- $C_{(a-v)}O_2$ reflects cardiac output's response to tissue O_2 needs.
- Clinical reference and derived values for pulmonary artery blood gases are affected by many pulmonary and cardiac related factors.
- Changes in $C_{(a-v)}O_2$ are early warning signs of cardiovascular decompensation.
- In patients who have normal, stable temperatures and who are not exhibiting excessive muscle use, VO_2 can be considered a constant.
- Due to intrapulmonary shunting, P_aO_2 affects $C_{(a-v)}O_2$.
- As $C_{(a-v)}O_2$ increases, $C_{\bar{v}}O_2$ and $S_{\bar{v}}O_2$ decrease.
- Hypoxia secondary to increased intrapulmonary shunt can be compensated for by increased $\dot{Q}_T$.
- Increased $\dot{Q}_T$ decreases $C_{(a-v)}O_2$, thus increasing $C_{\bar{v}}O_2$ and $S_{\bar{v}}O_2$.
- The oxygen extraction ratio (OER) expresses the amount of oxygen extracted as a percent of oxygen content.
- Normal OER is 25%.
- OER greater than 25% results from either inadequate C_aO_2 or inadequate $\dot{Q}_T$ to meet metabolic needs.
- Mixed venous oxygen saturation ($S_{\bar{v}}O_2$) equals oxygen delivered (DO_2) less the oxygen extracted ($C_{(a-v)}O_2$).
- With P_aO_2 greater than 60 mmHg, DO_2 is almost entirely a function of $\dot{Q}_T$ and the hemoglobin content of the blood.
- P_aO_2s greater than 100 mmHg add little to the DO_2 because of the shape of the oxyhemoglobin dissociation curve.
- On the steep part of the dissociation curve, large volumes of oxygen can be added to desaturated blood with little change in P_aO_2.
- The very forces that increase hemoglobin - oxygen affinity in the steep part of the curve also seek to prevent the release of oxygen at the tissue level.
- Extravascular fluid (EVF) volume exceeds the blood volume of the systemic capillaries by 5-10 times.
- Because EVF has no hemoglobin, the volume of oxygen in EVF is limited by the venous capillary PO_2 ($P_{\bar{v}}CO_2$).
- Increasing P_aO_2 from 60 mmHg to 100 mmHg makes little difference in the venous capillary PO_2.
- P_aO_2s from 200-300 mmHg also have little effect on venous capillary PO_2.
- P_aO_2s greater than 60 mmHg have little impact on oxygen extraction.

Tables

Measure	*Normal Range*
$P_{\bar{v}}O_2$	40 mmHg
$P_{\bar{v}}CO_2$	44 - 46 mmHg
pH	7.34 - 7.36
$C_{(a-v)}O_2$	5 ml/dL

Table 1: Mixed venous blood gas normal values.

Value	*Normal Range*
VO_2	250 ml/min (70 kilo subject)
$C_{(a-v)}O_2$	5 ml/dL
C_aO_2	20 ml/dL
$C_{\bar{v}}O_2$	15 ml/dL
OER	25%
DO_2	1,000 ml/min

Table 2: Normals for derived values.

Formulas

Arterial to Venous Oxygen Content Difference ($C_{(a-v)}O_2$)

$$C_{(a-v)}O_2 = C_aO_2 - C_{\bar{v}}O_2$$

Oxygen Consumption (VO_2)

$$VO_2 = C_{(a-v)}O_2 \times \dot{Q}_T \times 10$$

or

$$VO_2 = (C_IO_2 - C_EO_2)/\text{Minute}$$

Oxygen Extraction Ratio (OER)

$$OER = \frac{C_{(a-v)}O_2}{C_aO_2}$$

Oxygen Delivery (DO_2)

$$DO_2 = (C_aO_2 \times 10) \times \dot{Q}_T$$

Mixed Venous Oxygen Saturation

$$S_{\bar{v}}O_2 \simeq \frac{DO_2 - C_{(a-v)}O_2}{DO_2}$$

Problems

Select and mark the best answer.

1. The amount of oxygen utilized by the tissues can be determined by which of the following means?
   a. P_aO_2
   b. $C_{(a-v)}O_2$
   c. P_AO_2
   d. $S_{\bar{v}}O_2$
   e. HbO_2

2. Which of the following statements is true?
   a. Oxygen extraction usually exceeds oxygen carrying capacity.
   b. $P_aO_2 > P_{\bar{v}}O_2 > S_{\bar{v}}O_2$.
   c. $C_{(a-v)}O_2$ usually changes before P_aO_2.
   d. Increased pulmonary shunting increases VO_2.
   e. All of the above are correct.

3. For any given VO_2
   a. $C_{(a-v)}O_2$ varies inversely with cardiac output ($\dot{Q}_T$).
   b. $C_{(a-v)}O_2$ varies directly with cardiac output ($\dot{Q}_T$).
   c. $C_{(a-v)}O_2$ is not affected by cardiac output ($\dot{Q}_T$).
   d. $C_{(a-v)}O_2$ varies independently with VO_2.
   e. $C_{(a-v)}O_2$ is related to the endtidal PCO_2.

4. The most direct measure of oxygen extraction is the
   a. blood glucose level.
   b. endtidal CO_2 level.
   c. $P_aO_2 - P_AO_2$ value.
   d. $C_{(a-v)}O_2$ value.
   e. $S_{\bar{v}}O_2 - P_{\bar{v}}O_2$ value.

5. Which of the following is the "normal" value for $P_{\bar{v}}O_2$?
   a. 100 mmHg
   b. 40 mmHg
   c. 60 mmHg
   d. 0.6 mmHg
   e. 85 mmHg

6. The oxygen extraction ratio expresses the amount of oxygen removed from the arterial blood. In which unit is this value expressed?
   a. Liters/kilogram (L/K)
   b. Milligrams % (mg/100 ml)
   c. Grams/meter^2 (gm/m^2)
   d. Milliliters/decaliter (ml/dL)
   e. Percent (%)

7. Optimum biologic balance refers to
   a. increasing desired (good) metabolic outcomes.
   b. decreasing undesirable (bad) metabolic outcomes.
   c. hemostasis.
   d. All of the above are correct.
   e. Both a and b are correct.

8. Given the following data, select the correct information and calculate the oxygen extraction ratio: $P_{\bar{v}}O_2$ 47 mmHg, $C_{\bar{v}}O_2$ 18 ml/dL, $C_{(a-v)}O_2$ 6 ml/dL, C_aO_2 24 ml/dL, S_aO_2 98%, $P_{\bar{v}}CO_2$ 46 mmHg.
   a. 19%
   b. 25%
   c. 28%
   d. 30%
   e. 33%

9. Which of the following is the correct equation for calculating DO_2?
   a. $C_aO_2 \times \dot{Q}_T \times 10$.
   b. $C_aO_2/\dot{Q}_T \times 10$.
   c. $C_{(a-v)}O_2/VO_2$.
   d. $VO_2 \times 60/OER$.
   e. $\dot{Q}_T - VO_2$

10. Given a P_aO_2 of 65 mmHg and S_aO_2 of 92%, which of the following statements is correct?
    a. As $\dot{Q}_T$ increases C_aO_2 falls.
    b. Oxygen carrying capacity is pH dependent.
    c. P_aCO_2 will rise faster than P_aO_2.
    d. DO_2 is a function of [Hb] and $\dot{Q}_T$.
    e. All of the above are correct.

11. If $C_{(a-v)}O_2$ increases, this indicates that
    a. C_aO_2 may have decreased.
    b. less oxygen is being extracted.
    c. more oxygen is being extracted.
    d. $C_{\bar{v}}O_2$ may have increased.
    e. Both a and c are correct.

12. $S_{\bar{v}}O_2$ is
    a. directly dependent on $C_{(a-v)}O_2$.
    b. independent of $C_{(a-v)}O_2$.
    c. inversely dependent on $C_{(a-v)}O_2$.
    d. the same thing as $C_{(a-v)}O_2$.
    e. related to but not dependent on $C_{(a-v)}O_2$.

Answers to Problems

1. b: $C_{(a-v)}O_2$ is called the arterial to venous oxygen content difference. The oxygen which makes up the difference between that measured in artery (a) and that measured in mixed venous blood (v) consists of oxygen

taken up by the tissues for use in metabolic processes within the cells.

2. c: The $C_{(a\text{-}v)}O_2$ is a very sensitive indicator of cellular oxygen demand. As cells need more or less oxygen, the difference between the arterial and venous blood oxygen content varies rapidly. Adjustments in P_aO_2 take longer to accomplish than do changes in oxygen extraction.

3. a: At any given VO_2, as cardiac output ($\dot{Q}_T$) rises, the $C_{(a\text{-}v)}O_2$ will fall and vice versa. Since $VO_2 = C_{(a\text{-}v)}O_2 \times \dot{Q}_T \times 10$, if we keep VO_2 constant, any change in $C_{(a\text{-}v)}O_2$ will result in a change in the opposite direction for $\dot{Q}_T$.

4. d: The amount of oxygen extracted from arterial blood for use by the tissues can be best determined by measuring the amount of oxygen carried by a specific volume of arterial blood and comparing that with the volume of oxygen carried by blood which represents the average venous sample. The average venous sample will contain both oxygen saturated blood (from anatomical or physiologic shunts) and oxygen desaturated blood from tissue uptake. Thus we must measure the content of arterial blood (C_aO_2) and that of mixed venous blood ($C_{\bar{v}}O_2$). By combining like symbols (the distributive law) we get $C_{(a\text{-}v)}O_2$.

5. b: The "normal" value for venous oxygen tension ($P_{\bar{v}}O_2$) is 40 mmHg when breathing room air.

6. e: The oxygen extraction ratio expresses the amount of oxygen removed from the arterial blood by the tissues as a function of the arterial oxygen content. By analyzing the units of the measures from which the ratio is derived, we can determine the units appropriate to the OER.

   $OER = C_{(a\text{-}v)}O_2/C_aO_2$

   $C_{(a\text{-}v)}O_2$ is expressed in ml/dL

   C_aO_2 is expressed in ml/dL

   Since both units cancel, the ratio is unitless and is expressed as a decimal fraction or as a percentage.

7. d: Optimum biological activity is a concept which expresses the balance between good or useful biological activity (energy production) and the bad or damaging effects (oxygen toxicity) of metabolic processes. The aim is to minimize the bad effects while maximizing the good outcomes. This is sometimes called the min-max principle.

8. b: The oxygen extraction ratio (OER) = $C_{(a\text{-}v)}O_2/C_aO_2$

   $C_{(a\text{-}v)}O_2 = 6$ ml/dL

   $C_aO_2 = 24$ ml/dL

   $C_{(a\text{-}v)}O_2/C_aO_2 = 6$ ml/dL/24 ml/dL = 0.25 or 25%

9. a: DO_2 equals the amount of oxygen delivered to the tissues in one minute. The arterial oxygen content (C_aO_2) in ml/dL of blood expresses the amount of oxygen carried per 100 milliliters of blood; by multiplying that value by 10 we can determine the amount of oxygen carried per liter of blood. If we then multiply by the amount of blood circulated in one minute (the cardiac output: $\dot{Q}_T$), we can determine how much oxygen is carried (delivered) to the tissues in one minute.

10. d: When P_aO_2 exceeds 60 mmHg and S_aO_2 exceeds 90%, the delivery of oxygen to the cells (tissues) is dependent on the hemoglobin concentration and the cardiac output. Low levels of hemoglobin (anemia) or species of dysfunctional hemoglobin reduce the oxygen content, therefore reducing oxygen delivery. Changes in $\dot{Q}_T$ will bring either more or less blood past deoxygenated tissues (high or low volume states) or will change the rate at which blood passes the tissue (high or low flow states); in either case if the oxygen tension (pressure) in the extravascular fluid blood is higher than that of the arterial blood, oxygen exchange will not take place.

11. e: The interplay of two factors may cause $C_{(a\text{-}v)}O_2$ to increase; either the C_aO_2 has decreased while $C_{\bar{v}}O_2$ has remained constant or the $C_{\bar{v}}O_2$ has increased while the C_aO_2 remained unchanged or both have changed disproportionately.

12. a: Changes in $C_{(a\text{-}v)}O_2$ will have a direct but inverse effect on the $S_{\bar{v}}O_2$. As $C_{(a\text{-}v)}O_2$ increases, $S_{\bar{v}}O_2$ will fall; if $C_{(a\text{-}v)}O_2$ decreases, $S_{\bar{v}}O_2$ should rise. All of this assumes adequate arterial oxygenation.

Application Exercises

Situation 1

Jason Charles is a 24-year-old who was admitted to the ICU immediately after surgery three days ago. He was intubated and on a ventilator for the first post-op day, after which he was weaned and extubated. Today he is in acute respiratory distress and has a loose cough which is productive of large amounts of thick yellow secretions. Breath sounds are markedly decreased in all lung fields. His chest x-ray indicates a 5 lobe infiltrate. He is febrile with a temperature of 102° F. He is confused and disoriented.

ABGs reveal the following values: P_aO_2 120 mmHg, P_aCO_2 54, S_aO_2 99+ mmHg, F_IO_2 70%.

1. Is his F_IO_2 adequate?

2. What data do we need to assess tissue oxygenation?

3. What rationale do we have for reintubating Jason?

4. If Jason's hemoglobin is normal, what effect will decreased $\dot{Q}_T$ have on his $C_{(a-v)}O_2$?

Situation 2

You are in charge of setting up a hemodynamics/pulmonary physiology laboratory.

1. What is the minimum basic equipment you need in order to perform $C_{(a-v)}O_2$ determination?

2. What procedures do you need to perform to gather the appropriate data to estimate tissue oxygenation?

3. Your administrator asks you to explain the value of assessing oxygen content when we already have a blood gas lab. What is your reply?

Suggested Additional Readings

Bates, DV, *Respiratory Function,* 3rd edition, W.B. Saunders, Philadelphia, PA, 1989, pp. 52-54.

Madama, VC, *Pulmonary Function Testing and Cardiopulmonary Stress Testing,* Delmar Publishers, Albany, NY, 1993, pp. 200-246.

Marino, PL, *The ICU Book*, Lea & Febiger, Philadelphia, PA, 1991, pp. 14-22.

Stillwell, SB and Randall, EMc, *Pocket Guide to Cardiovascular Care*, C.V. Mosby, St. Louis, MO, 1990, pp. 99-101, 135-144.

CHAPTER 9

Assessment of Deadspace Ventilation

Objectives

After reading Chapter 9 and successfully completing this chapter of the workbook the student will be able to:

1. Describe deadspace ventilation.
2. Define the following terms:

acute pulmonary embolus	MV
alveolar deadspace	qualitative
anatomic deadspace	quantitative
control	respired gas (volume)
deadspace	synergistic
deadspace ventilation	three zone model
disparity	veno-arterial shunting
embolic phenomenon	$\dot{V}_E$
endtidal PCO_2	$\dot{V}_D$
F_ECO_2	$\dot{V}_A$
gravity-dependent	Volume preset ventilator
multiplicative	

3. Discuss the limitations of the current indirect methods of assessing deadspace ventilation.
4. Explain the subdivisions of exhaled ventilation ($\dot{V}_E$).
5. Discuss the relationship between $\dot{V}_A$ and $\dot{V}_D$.
6. Name the components of $\dot{V}_D$ and explain their relationship.
7. State the normal value for anatomic deadspace (V_{Danat}) per pound and per kilogram of body weight.
8. State the major causes of rapid shallow breathing leading to increased anatomic deadspace.
9. State the cause of alveolar deadspace (V_{Dalv}).
10. Define alveolar deadspace (V_{Dalv}).
11. State the three causes of arterial deadspace following pulmonary embolism.
12. Discuss the effect of the regional redistribution of pulmonary blood flow on the three-zone lung model.
13. Describe the effect of acute pulmonary hypertension on pulmonary blood distribution.
14. Discuss the effect of positive pressure ventilation (PPV) on deadspace ventilation.
15. Discuss the use of positive end expiratory pressure (PEEP) on $\dot{V}/Q$.
16. Name the three analytical methods of assessing $\dot{V}_D$.
17. Discuss the possible causes of increased minute ventilation (MV) when P_aCO_2 remains constant.
18. Discuss the reasons why P_aCO_2 is not considered a quantitative measure of alveolar ventilation ($\dot{V}_A$).
19. State three assumptions which allow for the substitution of MV for $\dot{V}_A$ when assessing ventilation.
20. Explain the clinical importance of an increasing MV to P_aCO_2 disparity.
21. Using a normal CO_2 exhalation curve, indicate the three phases of exhalation.
22. State the normal $[P_aCO_2 - P_ACO_2]$ value.
23. Given appropriate data, calculate $\dot{V}_D/V_T$ ratios.
24. Cite the four factors on which the accuracy of the calculations of the $\dot{V}_D/V_T$ ratios depends.
25. State the normal $\dot{V}_D/V_T$ range.
26. Describe the correct method of collecting a mean expired CO_2 sample.
27. Write the simplified clinical deadspace equation.
28. Describe the significance of the $\dot{V}_D/V_T$ ratio for the following observation: $\dot{V}_D/V_T = 0.4\text{-}0.6$ for ventilated and nonventilated patients.

Definitions

acute pulmonary embolism Sudden lodging of foreign material including blood clots in the pulmonary circulation.

alveolar deadspace (V_{Dalv}) An alveolus that is ventilated but not perfused. This gas volume reaches the alveoli but does not participate in gas exchange. Normal individuals do not have significant true alveolar deadspace because even the apical segments of the lung receive a small amount of perfusion.

anatomic deadspace (V_{Danat}) The gas remaining in the airway conducting structures at the end of each breath. This gas volume never reaches the alveoli and never participates in gas exchange. It approximates 1 ml/lb of ideal body weight.

control mode A method of mechanical ventilation in which the ventilator provides each breath at a predetermined frequency.

deadspace Areas of the lung that receive ventilation but do not have accompanying perfusion. This represents a high (infinite) $\dot{V}/\dot{Q}$ ratio.

deadspace ventilation The volume of inspired air which does not take part in gas exchange.

disparity The difference or gradient between two values.

embolic phenomenon A process by which emboli are produced and disseminated within the body.

endtidal PCO_2 The partial pressure of CO_2 in the final portion of expiration; this approximates the arterial P_aCO_2 and the P_ACO_2.

F_ECO_2 Mean fractional concentration of expired CO_2.

gravity-dependent areas of the lung The lung zones where the distribution of both perfusion and ventilation is the greatest. The gravity-dependent areas change according to the individual's body position. In the erect position, dependent lung regions are in the bases. In the supine position, dependent areas are located in the posterior aspects of the lung.

MV Minute ventilation; the total amount of gas moved into or out of the respiratory tract in one minute.

multiplicative A mathematical term describing a mathematical function requiring the multiplying together of two or more numbers. This may refer to simple multiplication, logarithmic or exponential calculations, or geometric progression.

qualitative How well something measures a factor and its presence (is it there?). This is a valuation or subjective measure.

quantitative How much of the substance is present; an objective (measurable) indicator.

respired gas (volume) The volume of gas that undergoes gas exchange (CO_2 for O_2) in the lungs.

synergistic An output response greater than expected from the input variable's characteristics (sometimes explained as the whole being greater than the sum of its parts).

three-zone model A conceptual model of the ventilation and perfusion relationships within the lung. In this model the lung is divided into three zones which can vary in size within the constraints of the total lung size. The zones are determined by the relative match of ventilation ($\dot{V}$) and perfusion ($\dot{Q}$).

Area	**$\dot{V}/\dot{Q}$**
Zone 1	$\dot{V} > \dot{Q}$
Zone 2	$\dot{V} \simeq \dot{Q}$
Zone 3	$\dot{V} < \dot{Q}$

veno-arterial shunting In the pulmonary system, unoxygenated blood from the pulmonary artery (venous blood) passes through the lung without encountering a ventilated alveoli and is mixed with oxygenated (arterial blood) in the pulmonary vein (arterial blood).

$\dot{V}_A$ Alveolar (respired) ventilation; ventilation going to the perfused alveoli.

$\dot{V}_D$ Deadspace ventilation; ventilation going to nonperfused areas of the respiratory tract.

$\dot{V}_D/\dot{V}_T$ Deadspace to tidal volume ratio, the proportion of the tidal volume which ventilated the deadspace in the respiratory tract.

$\dot{V}_E$ Exhaled ventilation, usually in liters/minute or milliliters/breath.

volume preset ventilator A mechanical ventilator which delivers a preset volume of gas to the patient.

Introduction

In this chapter Shapiro introduces us to the assessment of deadspace ventilation. He begins this discussion by defining and differentiating between various subcategories of deadspace ventilation.

Deadspace ventilation is first defined as an ever increasing high $\dot{V}/\dot{Q}$ unit which eventually ends as an "infinite" $\dot{V}/\dot{Q}$ unit. Shapiro indicates that although significant ventilation and oxygenation deficits can result from increased deadspace, it has no direct effect on respiration. Also noted is the point that ABGs offer no direct quantifiable method of assessing deadspace ventilation. Additionally, Shapiro notes that the current indirect methods of using blood gas data to predict deadspace are inaccurate and misapplied.

Exhaled ventilation volume ($\dot{V}_E$) is divided into two major components: respired gas ($\dot{V}_A$) and nonrespired gas ($\dot{V}_D$). The $\dot{V}_D$ is further subdivided into alveolar deadspace ventilation (V_{Dalv}) and anatomic deadspace ventilation (V_{Danat}). Anatomic deadspace is essentially fixed (1 ml/lb or 2.2 ml/kg). Therefore, changes in deadspace at fixed $\dot{V}_E$ can result only from changes in (V_{Dalv}). As V_{Dalv} changes, concurrent changes occur in work of breathing (WOB) due to the reduced ability to effect O_2/CO_2 exchange. Anatomical deadspace can increase during shallow, rapid breathing, during increased work of breathing secondary to decreased compliance, or with central nervous system dysfunction.

Alveolar deadspace refers to nonperfused but ventilated alveolar spaces. These volumes are affected by both embolic phenomena and pulmonary perfusion deficits caused by hemodynamic redistribution. Among the sequela of pulmonary emboli are venous to arterial shunting, decreased $\dot{V}/\dot{Q}$ and increased work of breathing, all of which lead to arterial hypoxemia.

Using West's Three-Zone Model of the lung as an index, Shapiro next discusses the effects of regional distribution of pulmonary blood flow and decreased cardiac output on the magnitude of lung zones. Acute reduction of cardiac output will cause increases in the bounds of Zones 1 and 2 secondary to reduced pulmonary perfusion pressure. Decreased mixed venous oxygen content adds to the hypoxemia associated with the acute decrease in cardiac output. Acute pulmonary hypertension is commonly caused by acidemia, decreased alveolar oxygen tension and severe arterial hypoxemia.

Shapiro next discusses the redistribution of ventilation as a cause of increased deadspace. Using the example of positive airway pressure therapy, he discusses the fact that positive pressure tends to selectively favor ventilation of nongravity-dependent lung zones (Zone 1 and Zone 2). This results in increasing deadspace ventilation. Positive end expiratory pressure (PEEP) may increase both ventilation and perfusion of alveolar deadspace units.

There are, according to Shapiro, three clinically useful methods of assessing deadspace ventilation: minute ventilation (MV) to P_aCO_2 disparity; a-A PCO_2 gradient; and deadspace to tidal volume ratio ($\dot{V}_D/V_T$). Minute volume changes without concurrent changes in P_aCO_2 indicate a change in either $\dot{V}_D$ or CO_2 production. Shapiro holds that P_aCO_2 is not a quantitative measure of alveolar ventilation ($\dot{V}_A$). P_aCO_2 is, however, grossly qualitative of minute ventilation if: (a) the anatomic deadspace is normal and changes proportionately with the minute ventilation, (b) P_aCO_2 is near 40 mmHg, and (c) CO_2 production is normal. Given these conditions, MV - P_aCO_2 qualitates the presence of acute deadspace-producing conditions. In other words, you can determine the presence of the condition but not its extent.

The a-A CO_2 endtidal gradient normally varies by less than 2 mmHg. The comparison of "a," the arterial carbon dioxide tension (P_aCO_2) which is an index of CO_2 production, and "A," the partial pressure of endtidal carbon dioxide ($P_{et}CO_2$) which indicates CO_2 elimination, provides an indication of the relative amount of deadspace. Acute changes in the a-A CO_2 gradient signal increases in deadspace ventilation. To be a useful measure, baseline data is needed from which trends can be projected.

The technique of $\dot{V}_D/V_T$ ratio analysis is Shapiro's next and main method of determining the extent of deadspace ventilation. A major factor affecting the accuracy of the ratio analysis is the collection of gas samples to analyze for F_ECO_2. Shapiro stresses four prerequisites for good sample collection. First, the patient must have a reasonably normal and stable ventilatory pattern. Next, the patient's metabolic rate must be relatively normal. Third, there must be essentially normal cardiovascular function. Last, the proper gas sampling procedures must be carried out.

Please note that multiple variations in the above factors may result in incorrect data due to the additive (synergistic) effects of mathematical coupling. That is, an error of size 2 in factor A and an error of size 3 in factor B may be offsetting, additive or multiplicative on the whole system (A + B). An illustration is given below:

Effect Type	Error A	Error B	Error A + B
Additive	2	3	5
Offsetting	2	3	1
Multiplicative	2	3	6

Sample collection time varies from 5-10 minutes for spontaneously breathing subjects to 23 minutes for patients on mechanical ventilation in the control mode. A normal spontaneously breathing patient has a $\dot{V}_D/V_T$ ratio of 0.2 to 0.4 (20-40%). To calculate $\dot{V}_D/V_T$ the following relationships are highlighted:

$$\dot{V}_E = \dot{V}_A + \dot{V}_D$$

F_ECO_2 = CO_2 volume collected/total volume collected (F_ECO_2 = Fraction of mean expired CO_2)

The volume of expired CO_2 must come from either the alveolar volume ($\dot{V}_A$) or the deadspace volume ($\dot{V}_D$):

$$\dot{V}_E \times (F_ECO_2) = (\dot{V}_A \times F_ACO_2) + (\dot{V}_D \times F_DCO_2) \text{ but:}$$

$$\dot{V}_DCO_2 \times F_DCO_2 \simeq 0 \text{ so:}$$

$$\dot{V}_E \times (F_ECO_2) \simeq (\dot{V}_A \times F_ACO_2) \text{ and:}$$

$$\dot{V}_A = \dot{V}_A - \dot{V}_D \text{ thus:}$$

extending the formula and dividing each side by F_ECO_2 and V_E we get:

$$\dot{V}_D/V_T = \frac{F_ACO_2 - F_ECO_2}{F_ACO_2}$$

Realizing that the P_ACO_2 is proportional to the F_ECO_2, that P_ACO_2 is $\simeq$ P_aCO_2, and that V_T $\simeq$ $\dot{V}_A$ we can further simplify the equation to its final form:

$$\dot{V}_D/V_T = \frac{P_aCO_2 - P_ECO_2}{P_aCO_2}$$

This formula indicates that as deadspace increases in proportion to the tidal volume, the P_aCO_2 will decrease.

In patients on controlled mechanical ventilators, a 5 liter expired gas sample is equivalent to a 5-10 minute sample from a spontaneously breathing subject. $\dot{V}_D/V_T$ greater than 0.8 suggests a significant deadspace increase. In patients on control mode ventilation, the normal $\dot{V}_D/V_T$ is 0.4-0.6.

Key Points

- $\dot{V}/\dot{Q}$ ratio ranges from zero $\dot{V}/\dot{Q}$ (shunt units) to infinite $\dot{V}/\dot{Q}$ (deadspace units).

- Deadspace has no direct effect on respiration, although clinically significant oxygenation and ventilation deficits can result in increased deadspace.
- Arterial blood gases are not reliable, quantifiable indicators of increased deadspace.
- Current indirect methods of using ABGs to assess deadspace are imprecise and often misused.
- Exhaled ventilatory volume ($\dot{V}_E$) consists of alveolar ventilation ($\dot{V}_A$) and deadspace ventilation ($\dot{V}_D$).
- $\dot{V}_A$ is respired gas; $\dot{V}_D$ is unrespired gas.
- Increased $\dot{V}_D$ requires increased $\dot{V}_E$ if $\dot{V}_A$ is to remain adequate for metabolic needs.
- The need to increase $\dot{V}_E$ results in an increase in the work of breathing (WOB).
- $\dot{V}_D$ consists of anatomic deadspace, V_{Danat}, and alveolar deadspace, V_{Dalv}.
- Normal V_{Danat} equals 1 ml/pound or 2.2 ml/kilogram of body weight.
- V_{Danat} is usually stable.
- The major cause of increased V_{Danat} is rapid, shallow breathing due to increased WOB secondary to decreased pulmonary compliance and/or CNS dysfunction.
- V_{Dalv} results from infinite $\dot{V}/\dot{Q}$ units (ventilated but not perfused alveoli) secondary to embolism and perfusion redistribution in the lungs.
- Distal pulmonary circulation can be blocked by blood clots or other substances which occlude a branch of the pulmonary arteries.
- Blocked distal capillaries result in unperfused but ventilated alveoli, leading to alveolar deadspace-producing disease.
- An expected outcome of pulmonary emboli is arterial hypoxemia. This is due to venous to arterial shunting (decreased $\dot{V}/\dot{Q}$ matching) and increased WOB.
- Acute decreases in cardiac output increase Zone 2 and Zone 3 lung areas by decreasing pulmonary perfusion pressure. This lowers perfusion in the nongravity-dependent lung zones.
- Hypoxemia related to decreased cardiac output occurs primarily due to decreased mixed venous oxygen content ($C_{(a-v)}O_2$).
- When deadspace increases, clinicians must evaluate work of breathing.
- Acute pulmonary hypertension is a common cause of pulmonary perfusion redistribution.
- Increased vascular resistance in acute pulmonary hypertension causes increased perfusion to the gravity-dependent portions of the lungs, Zones 2 and 3.
- Among the causes of acute pulmonary hypertension are acidosis, low P_aO_2 and severe arterial hypoxemia.
- Redistribution of ventilation can create deadspace ventilation without either causing or affecting perfusion distribution.
- Positive pressure ventilation (PPV) preferentially augments ventilation to nongravity-dependent portions of the lung without increasing cardiac output, thereby increasing deadspace ventilation.
- PEEP (positive end expiratory pressure) often improves $\dot{V}/\dot{Q}$.
- There are three clinically available methods for assessing $\dot{V}_D$: MV to P_aCO_2 disparity, a-A PCO_2 gradient and $\dot{V}_D/V_T$ ratio.
- Failure to decrease P_aCO_2 with increased MV results in MV to P_aCO_2 disparity (CO_2 is not changed proportionately to MV), indicating increased deadspace ventilation.
- $MV = \dot{V}_A + \dot{V}_D$.
- If MV increases without proportional changes in P_aCO_2, either CO_2 production has increased or deadspace ventilation has increased.
- In normal individuals, as MV changes, P_aCO_2 changes in the opposite direction in a nonlinear (hyperbolic) manner.
- P_aCO_2 is a qualitative measure of the adequacy of alveolar ventilation and a true reflection of the alveolar CO_2 but is not a quantitative measure of alveolar ventilation.
- Assuming that V_{Danat} is normal and changes proportionately with the MV, P_aCO_2 is approximately 40 mmHg and CO_2 production is normal, $\dot{V}_A$ will approximate MV.
- MV to P_aCO_2 disparity $\simeq$ $\dot{V}_A$ to P_aCO_2 disparity.
- MV to P_aCO_2 disparity is, under ideal conditions, a qualitative index of the status of $\dot{V}_D$ in acute disease processes.
- The a-A PCO_2 gradient is normally less than 2 mmHg.
- Acute increases in a-A PCO_2 indicate increased deadspace ventilation.
- Trend analysis of a-A PCO_2 is an excellent monitoring tool.
- The deadspace to tidal volume ration ($\dot{V}_D/V_T$) is the classic measure of deadspace status.

- $\dot{V}_D/V_T$ accuracy depends on a stable, consistent respiratory pattern, "normal" metabolic rate, adequate cardiovascular function, and procedural and technical competence in the collection and analysis of the gas sample.
- Gas sample collection time ranges from 5-10 minutes for spontaneously breathing subjects to a 1- to 2-minute (5 liter) sample in the subject being controlled on a volume ventilator.
- As $\dot{V}_D$ increases, more dilution of P_ACO_2 occurs. In other words, the larger the proportion of deadspace in each breath, the less the proportion of CO_2 in the expired gas.
- $\dot{V}_D/V_T$ increases to greater than 0.4 in PPV patients due to increased $\dot{V}_D$. Normal $\dot{V}_D/V_T$ range in PPV patients is 0.4-0.6 (40-60%).
- $\dot{V}_D/V_T$ ratios greater than 0.8 in PPV patients indicate a significant increase in deadspace ventilation.
- Normal $\dot{V}_D/V_T$ ratio equals 0.2-0.4 (20-49%).
- $\dot{V}_E = \dot{V}_A + \dot{V}_D$.
- $\dot{V}_E$ = expired gas; $\dot{V}_A$ = respired gas; $\dot{V}_D$ = nonrespired gas ($\dot{V}_D = V_{Dalv} + V_{Danat}$).
- The mean expired fraction of CO_2 (F_ECO_2) is the average fractional concentration of CO_2 in an expired gas sample.
- $F_ECO_2 = \dfrac{\text{Volume expired } CO_2 \text{ collected}}{\text{Volume total expired gas collected}}$
- Since $\dot{V}_A$ has both alveolar (V_{Dalv}) and anatomic (V_{Danat}) deadspace components, F_ECO_2 equals $\dot{V}_E \times F_ECO_2 (\dot{V}_A \times F_ACO_2) + (\dot{V}_D \times F_DCO_2)$
- but $(\dot{V}_D \times F_DCO_2) \simeq 0$
- Dropping $(\dot{V}_D \times F_DCO_2)$
  $\dot{V}_E \times F_ECO_2 = (\dot{V}_A \times F_ACO_2)$
- and $\dot{V}_A = \dot{V}_E - \dot{V}_D$
- Substituting for $\dot{V}_A$:
  $\dot{V}_E \times F_ECO2 = (\dot{V}_E - \dot{V}_D) \times F_ACO_2)$
  or
  $(\dot{V}_D \times F_ACO_2) = (\dot{V}_E \times F_ACO_2) - (\dot{V}_E \times F_ECO_2)$.
- Dividing each side of the equation to cancel common terms ($\dot{V}_E$ and F_ACO_2) we get:
  $$\frac{\dot{V}_D}{V_T} = \frac{F_ACO_2 - F_ECO_2}{F_ACO_2}$$
- However, $F_ACO_2 \simeq P_ACO_2$, $P_ACO_2 \simeq P_aCO_2$, $V_T \simeq \dot{V}_D$ thus:
  $$\frac{\dot{V}_D}{V_T} = \frac{P_ACO_2 - P_ECO_2}{P_ACO_2}$$

Formulas

Minute Ventilation

$\dot{V}_E = \dot{V}_A + \dot{V}_D$ or $MV = \dot{V}_A + \dot{V}_D$

Deadspace Ventilation

$\dot{V}_D = V_{Danat} + V_{Dalv}$

Arterial to Alveolar CO_2 Disparity

$P_aCO_2 - P_ACO_2 = (a\text{-}A)PCO_2$

Tidal Volume to Deadspace Ratio

$$\frac{\dot{V}_D}{V_T}$$

Calculated F_ECO_2

$$F_ECO_2 = \frac{\text{volume of } CO_2 \text{ collected}}{\text{total gas volume collected}}$$

Calculation of $\dot{V}_D$

$(\dot{V}_E \times F_ECO_2) = (\dot{V}_A \times F_ACO_2) + (\dot{V}_D \times F_DCO_2)$

but: $(\dot{V}_D \times F_DCO_2) \simeq 0$

therefore: $(\dot{V}_E \times F_ECO_2) = (\dot{V}_A \times F_ACO_2)$

$\dot{V}_A = \dot{V}_E - \dot{V}_D$ thus:

$\dot{V}_E \times F_ECO_2 = (\dot{V}_E - \dot{V}_D) \times (F_ACO_2)$; rearranging:

$\dot{V}_D(F_ACO_2) = \dot{V}_A(F_ACO_2) \times F_ECO_2 - \dot{V}_E$

Dividing each side of the equation by F_ACO_2 and V_E:

$$\frac{\dot{V}_D}{\dot{V}_E} = \frac{F_ACO_2 - F_ECO_2}{F_ACO_2}$$

$F_ACO_2 \simeq P_aCO_2$ and
$F_ECO_2 \simeq P_ECO_2$ and
$\dot{V}_E \simeq V_T$

therefore: $\dot{V}_D = \dfrac{P_aCO_2 - P_ECO_2}{P_aCO_2}$

Tables and Figures

MV ≃ V_{alv} if:
- V_{Danat} is normal.
- V_{Danat} changes proportionately with MV.
- P_aCO_2 is not significantly greater than 40 mmHg.
- CO_2 production is close to normal.

Table 1: Relationship of MV to $\dot{V}_A$.

$\dot{V}_D/V_T$ is useful when:
- the respiratory pattern is reasonably constant.
- metabolic rate is relatively normal.
- cardiovascular function is close to normal.
- correct technical procedures are used for gas sample acquisition and analysis.

Table 2: Factors affecting quality of $\dot{V}_D/V_T$ data.

Variable		*Value*
a-A PCO_2		2 mmHg
$\dot{V}_D/V_T$ ratio	Spontaneous Breathing	< 0.2 - 0.4 (20 - 40%)
	Positive Press Ventilation	0.4 - 0.6 (40 - 60%)
	Significant $\dot{V}_D$ > on PPV	> 0.8 (> 80%)

Table 3: Normal values.

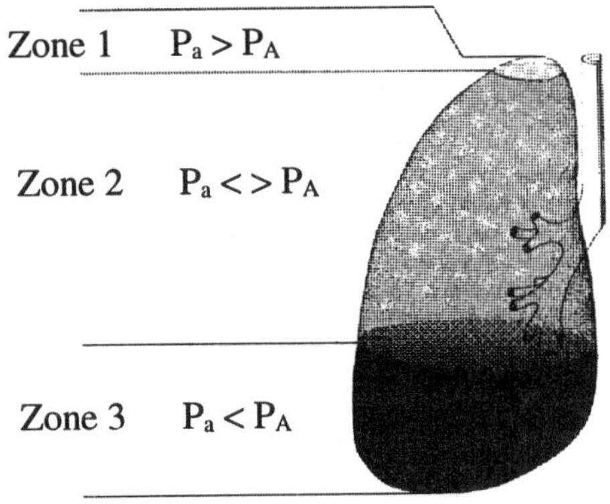

Figure 1: Three-zone model of the lung (upright).

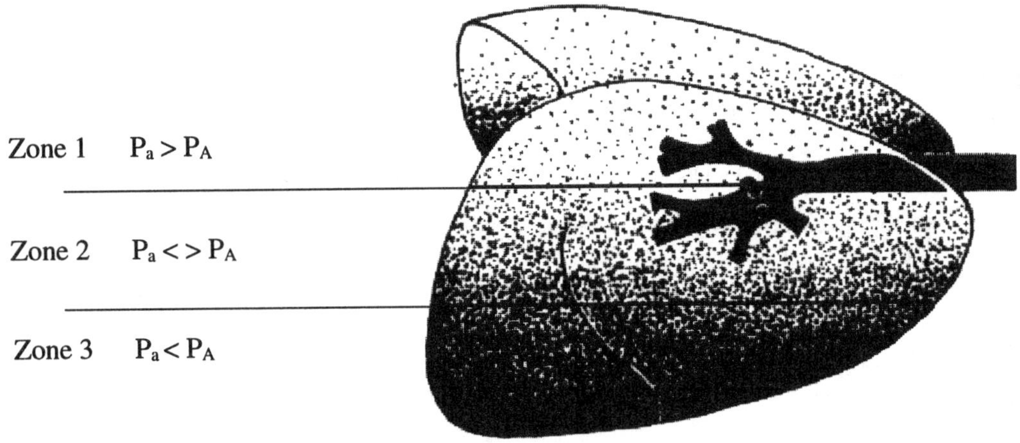

Figure 2: Three-zone model of the lung (supine).

Problems

Select and mark the best answer.

1. Which of the following is the most common cause for acutely increased deadspace ventilation ($\dot{V}_D$) ?
   a. Decreased P_aCO_2
   b. Acutely increased V_T
   c. Decreased F_IO_2
   d. Increased respiratory rate
   e. Acutely increased $\dot{Q}_T$

2. Which of the following are methods for assessing deadspace ventilation?
   I. $\dot{V}_D/V_T$
   II. a-A PO_2
   III. MV to P_aCO_2
   IV. a-A PCO_2
   V. $\dot{Q}_T/V_T$

   a. I and II
   b. I, III and IV
   c. II, III and V
   d. I, II and IV
   e. I only

3. The normal a-A PCO_2 value is
   a. 22 mmHg.
   b. 13 mmHg.
   c. 8 mmHg.
   d. 2 mmHg.
   e. 0 mmHg.

4. The normal $\dot{V}_D/V_T$ ratio range is
   a. 0.2-0.4 (20-40%).
   b. 0.1-0.2 (10-20%).
   c. 0.85-0.95 (85-95%).
   d. 0.3-0.5 (30-50%).
   e. 0.25-0.35 (25-35%).

5. Under which condition will collection of a mean expired gas sample for CO_2 analysis be most accurate and practical?
   a. Spontaneously breathing patient
   b. Patient on assist mode mechanical ventilation
   c. Patient on control mode mechanical ventilation
   d. Patient on mechanical ventilation with SIMV
   e. Patient on BiPAP

6. Which of the following represents the clinical deadspace equation?
   a. $\dot{V}_A = \dot{V}_D + V_T$
   b. $\dot{V}_E \times \dot{V}_D = V_T$
   c. $\dot{V}_D/V_T = (P_aCO_2 - P_ECO_2)/P_aCO_2$
   d. $\dot{V}_D = V_{Danat} \times V_{Dalv} - \dot{V}_E$
   e. $V_{Dtot} = \dot{V}_D \times$ Resp rate

7. What range of $\dot{V}_D/V_T$ indicates significant increases in deadspace ventilation in patients on positive pressure ventilation (PPV)?
   a. < 0.6
   b. > 0.8
   c. < 0.8
   d. 0.1-0.6
   e. 0.2-0.7

8. As $\dot{V}_D/V_T$ increases, what effects do you expect to see in $\dot{V}_D$ if $\dot{V}_E$ remains constant?
   a. $\dot{V}_D$ increases.
   b. $\dot{V}_D$ decreases.
   c. $\dot{V}_D$ remains constant.
   d. Both a and b are possible.
   e. None of the above should occur.

9. Given V_{Dalv} 60 ml, V_{Danat} 140 ml, and V_T 600 ml, what is the $\dot{V}_A$?
   a. 800 ml
   b. 740 ml
   c. 340 ml
   d. 400 ml
   e. 540 ml

10. The term *deadspace unit* refers to alveoli with
    a. low opening pressure.
    b infinite $\dot{V}/\dot{Q}$.
    c. zero $\dot{V}/\dot{Q}$.
    d. increased $\dot{V}_A$.
    e. alveolar wall rupture.

11. A shunt unit indicates
    a. increased V_T.
    b. tension pneumothorax.
    c. zero $\dot{V}/\dot{Q}$.
    d. infinite $\dot{V}/\dot{Q}$.
    e. decreased ventilation.

12. Which of the following best reflects the relationship between $\dot{V}_E$ and V_T?
    a. $\dot{V}_E \simeq V_T$.
    b. $\dot{V}_E = V_T$.
    c. $\dot{V}_E$ does not equal V_T.
    d. $\dot{V}_E$ and V_T are not related.
    e. $\dot{V}_E$ and $\dot{V}_A$ both equal V_T.

13. Given the following data, calculate the $\dot{V}_D/V_T$ ratio and determine its "normality" for a spontaneously breathing patient: V_T 560 ml, V_{Danat} 250 ml, V_{Dalv} 142 ml.

    a. Normal
    b. Low normal
    c. High normal
    d. Abnormally low
    e. Abnormally high

14. Which portion of V_T takes part in gas exchange?
   a. V_T
   b. $\dot{V}_A$
   c. V_{Danat}
   d. V_{Dalv}
   e. Both b and c are correct.

15. When using a sample collection bag to obtain gas samples for analysis of deadspace (F_ECO_2), what is the sampling time in spontaneously breathing subjects?
   a. 2-3 minutes
   b. < 2 minutes
   c. 5-6 minutes
   d. 7 minutes
   e. 5-10 minutes

Answers to Problems

1. e: When $\dot{Q}_T$ increases acutely, more blood perfuses non-ventilated alveolar units over a given period of time. This increases the probability that it will not "dump" its CO_2 load in the lung.

2. b: $\dot{V}_D/V_T$, MV to P_aCO_2 disparity, and a-A PCO_2 all either directly or indirectly examine the relationship of total inspired volume to the deadspace portion of that volume. a-A PO_2 examines oxygenation, not deadspace. $\dot{Q}_T/V_T$ is the respiratory exchange ratio equation.

3. d: P_ACO_2 closely approximates P_aCO_2, in part because of its high diffusion coefficient (20 × greater than O_2) and also because of the small distance between pulmonary capillaries and alveoli.

4. a: $\dot{V}_D$ is approximately 20-40% of the tidal volume. $\dot{V}_D$ is usually estimated to be about 1/3 of the tidal volume in clinical applications.

5. c: Patients on controlled ventilation have stable, predictable V_T and respiratory patterns. This provides a more uniform sample in a shorter period of time.

6. e: $\dot{V}_D/V_T = \dfrac{P_aCO_2 - P_ECO_2}{P_aCO_2}$, where $(P_aCO_2 - P_ECO_2)$ is the difference between the arterial and the mean expired PCO_2. Due to the diffusibility of CO_2, only deadspace influences the exchange of CO_2. Therefore, increases in the alveolar to arterial CO_2 indicate increased deadspace ventilation.

7. b: $\dot{V}_D/V_T$ normally equals 0.4-0.6 in PPV patients. A $\dot{V}_D/V_T$ greater than 0.8 represents a significant increase in $\dot{V}_D$ for PPV patients.

8. a: $V_T \simeq \dot{V}_E$; if $\dot{V}_E$ remains constant, then $\dot{V}_D$ must increase.
   Let $\dot{V}_E = 500$ ml; $\dot{V}_{D1} = 200$ ml; $\dot{V}_{D2} = 250$ ml.
   $\dot{V}_{D1}/V_T = 200/500 = 0.4$; $\dot{V}_{D2}/V_T = 250/500 = 0.5$

9. d: $\dot{V}_A = V_T - \dot{V}_D$; and $\dot{V}_D = (V_{Danat} + V_{Dalv})$ so:
   $\dot{V}_A = V_T - (V_{Danat} + V_{Dalv})$
   $\dot{V}_A = 600 - (60 + 140)$
   $\dot{V}_A = 600 - 200$
   $\dot{V}_A = 400$ ml

10. b: A deadspace unit has ventilated but not perfused alveoli. This represents wasted ventilation and increased work of breathing ($\dot{V} = 1$) ($\dot{Q} = 0$); $\dot{V}/\dot{Q} = 1/0 = 1$.

11. c: Shunt units don't have a match between ventilation and perfusion. These units are perfused but not ventilated ($\dot{V} = 0$) ($\dot{Q} = 1$); $\dot{V}/\dot{Q} = 0/1 = 0$.

12. a: $\dot{V}_E$ is approximately the same as V_T. Any differences relate to trapped volumes, O_2 uptake/CO_2 elimination variances, and/or H_2O vapor additions in the exhaled gas volume.

13. e: Normal range for $\dot{V}_D/V_T$ in mechanically ventilated subjects on PPV is 0.4-0.6. In this example the ratio is 0.7, indicating an abnormally high $\dot{V}_D/V_T$ ratio.

14. b: $V_T = \dot{V}_A + (V_{Dalv} + V_{Danat})$. $\dot{V}_D$ represents ventilated but not perfused portions of the pulmonary system. Only $\dot{V}_A$ ventilates areas of the lungs capable of respiration.

15. e: Due to variations between inhaled and exhaled volumes and variations in the breathing patterns of spontaneously breathing subjects, a relatively large sample is needed to determine F_ECO_2. Thus 5-10 minutes are required to obtain a sufficiently large sample and ensure adequate and accurate sampling.

Application Exercises

Situation 1

Terry Tyler is a 35-year-old, 75 kilogram RN admitted post-flu with a chief complaint of generalized pain and fatigue. Subsequent lab and radiologic tests confirmed the presence of an atypical mycosis. The mycosis was successfully treated, but the chemotherapeutic agents have decreased his immune response to a level where he has now contracted a pneumonic process in both lower lobes and the right middle lobe.

Terry is now in the ICU on 70% oxygen via partial rebreathing mask. During teaching rounds you are asked to address the following issues:

1. Describe and justify the appropriate patient position which will maximize $\dot{V}/\dot{Q}$ match in this patient.

2. Given the following data, calculate Terry's $\dot{V}_D/V_T$ ratio:
   P_aCO_2 48 mmHg, P_ECO_2 35 mmHg
   Is this a normal value for $\dot{V}_D/V_T$? For (a-A)PCO_2?

3. Using Dalton's Law as a model, explain why we can use P_ECO_2 as a substitute for F_ECO_2 in determining Terry's $\dot{V}_D/V_T$ ratio.

4. How would you determine the MV to P_aCO_2 disparity if Terry's minute volume (MV) equaled 9.0 liters when the above values were obtained?

Situation 2

Wesley Adams is a 27-year-old professional football player who is seen in the ER for evaluation of thoracic cage injuries received in yesterday's conference championship game (his team won). On the last play of the game Wes was hit by blockers on both sides of his chest. He says he heard a "popping" sound but experienced no pain at the time. Back at his hotel he noted deep bruising on the right lateral chest wall and began experiencing increasing shortness of breath and stabbing pains beneath the site of the bruise.

Physical examination revealed a well-developed male exhibiting guarding over the right lateral chest wall. The patient was tachypneic and complaining of shortness of breath and pain. Chest x-rays revealed fractures of the midribs and a collapsed and opaque right middle lobe which exhibited an intrapleural fluid level. Thoracentesis produced 350 ml of bloody fluid.

ABGs were obtained with the following results: pH 7.52, P_aCO_2 45 mmHg, P_aO_2 68 mmHg, F_IO_2 0.21.

1. Describe the results of Wes' injury with respect to: change in lung zones, shunt vs. deadspace ventilation and $\dot{V}_D/V_T$ ratio.

2. Why did Wes' pulmonary symptoms have a delayed appearance? Address this question in terms of the points outlined above.

3. Describe the sequence of events you would expect to note in terms of deadspace as Wes' condition resolves.

Suggested Additional Readings

Hall, JB, Schmidt, GA and Wood, LD, *Principles of Critical Care: Companion Handbook*, McGraw-Hill, Inc., 1993, pp. 104-109.

Scanlan, CL, Spearman, CB and Sheldon, RL, *Egan's Fundamentals of Respiratory Care,* 5th edition, C.V. Mosby, St. Louis, MO, 1990, pp.198-203.

Sproule, BJ, Lynne-Davies, P and King, EG, *Fundamentals of Respiratory Disease*, Churchill Livingstone, New York, NY, 1981, pp. 23-25.

Wilkins, RL, Sheldon, RL and Krider, SJ, *Clinical Assessment in Respiratory Care,* 2nd edition, C.V. Mosby, St. Louis, MO, 1990, pp. 76, 81, 191, 198-200.

Wilson, RF, *Critical Care Manual,* 2nd edition, F.A. Davis, Inc., Philadelphia, PA, 1992, pp. 372-373, 398-401.

CHAPTER 10

Deadspace- and Shunt-Producing Pathology

Objectives

After reading Chapter 10 and successfully completing this chapter of the workbook the student will be able to:

1. Define the term *deadspace ventilation.*
2. Define the term *intrapulmonary shunt.*
3. Identify the three types of deadspace-producing pathology.
4. Identify the three types of shunt-producing pathology.
5. Given a list of pathologic diseases or conditions, identify them as causes of deadspace or shunt.
6. Given a list of pathologic diseases or conditions, place them in the correct classification of deadspace or shunt.
7. In the presence of adequate cardiopulmonary reserve, describe blood gas alterations and cardiovascular responses in individuals with deadspace-producing pathology and shunt-producing pathology.
8. Compare the effects of oxygen therapy in individuals with deadspace-producing pathology with those with shunt-producing pathology.
9. Given a patient situation with shunt- or deadspace-producing pathology, identify the classic physiologic changes or response in the following:
   a. minute volume
   b. blood gas values
   c. cardiovascular system
   d. effect of oxygen therapy

Definitions

acute pulmonary embolism Sudden lodging of foreign material including blood clots in the pulmonary circulation.

alveolar deadspace (V_{Dalv}) An alveolus that is ventilated but not perfused. This gas volume reaches the alveoli but does not participate in gas exchange. Normal individuals do not have significant true alveolar deadspace because even the apical segments of the lung receive a small amount of perfusion.

anatomic deadspace (V_{Danat}) The gas remaining in the airway conducting structures at the end of each breath. This gas volume never reaches the alveoli and never participates in gas exchange. It approximates 1 ml/lb of ideal body weight.

cardiopulmonary reserve The actual ability of the cardiopulmonary system to maintain adequate function in the face of additional physiologic stress on the organism.

deadspace ventilation The volume of inspired air which does not take part in gas exchange.

embolus A foreign object such as a blood clot, air bubble, tissue or infected material that circulates in the bloodstream until it becomes lodged in a blood vessel. In a **pulmonary** embolus, it becomes lodged in a pulmonary artery, or arteriole. A single embolus or an embolic shower (many small emboli) may lodge in the lung's circulation.

intrapulmonary shunt That portion of the cardiac output entering the left side of the heart that does not have perfect gas exchange with perfect alveoli.

thrombophlebitis Inflammation of a vein which is often accompanied by the formation of a blood clot. Because of the presence of calf pain, the affected vein is likely to be a deep leg vein. The individual is usually put on strict bed rest and is observed for signs of pulmonary embolism or other complications.

work of breathing (WOB) Energy cost of breathing; how much energy is needed to move a given volume of gas through the ventilatory process.

Introduction

In Chapter 10 Shapiro applies the concepts of pulmonary physiology discussed in the previous chapters to a critical topic in respiratory medicine — deadspace- and shunt-producing pathology. This chapter provides clear guidelines for the reader to help identify those patients with increased deadspace and those with increased shunt.

Before continuing in the discussion of the chapter, a brief review of pathologic or clinical causes of deadspace and shunt is indicated. In Chapter 9 Shapiro identifies the three types of deadspace-producing pathology: anatomic, alveolar and ventilation in excess of perfusion.

Anatomic deadspace is affected by a few factors; e.g., lean body weight, posture, position of the neck and jaw, and the presence of artificial airways. Of all the possible causes, an increase in anatomic deadspace is usually the result of a *rapid, shallow breathing*. An individual's breathing pattern changes in response to one of two causes: first, rapid, shallow breathing is the adjustment individuals make to a reduction in lung compliance; and second, central nervous system abnormalities may affect individuals' breathing patterns.

The author separates the next two types of deadspace in order to clarify in the reader's mind that an increased deadspace may be secondary to a reduced or redistributed pulmonary perfusion (alveolar deadspace) or elevated or redistributed ventilation (ventilation in excess of perfusion). Both abnormalities cause a high ventilation/perfusion ratio, but the etiologies are very different.

Two primary causes of alveolar deadspace mentioned by the author are *acute pulmonary embolism* and *redistribution of pulmonary perfusion*. Acute pulmonary embolism is the classic example given as a cause of alveolar deadspace. A blood clot or another substance (e.g., infected material, fat globules or tumor material) lodges in the pulmonary artery or one of its branches and prevents perfusion past the point of obstruction. Since the alveoli are not involved, ventilation continues to the area of the lung that is not receiving blood flow. Hence, there is an increase in alveolar deadspace. A change in the regional distribution of pulmonary blood flow is the second cause of an increase in alveolar deadspace. A reduction in cardiac output (CO) or a sudden increase in pulmonary vascular resistance (PVR) will affect the distribution of pulmonary blood flow. A decrease in CO will reduce pulmonary perfusion pressure and the flow of blood to nongravity-dependent areas of the lung. This results in an increase in alveolar deadspace. Acute pulmonary hypertension increases the distribution of perfusion to the more gravity-dependent areas of the lung. The critical factor that really affects the alveolar deadspace is the reduction in right ventricular CO. This slight decrease in CO increases the alveolar deadspace.

Ventilation in excess of perfusion is the final type of deadspace-producing pathology. Shapiro identifies *alveolar septal destruction* and *positive pressure ventilation* as two examples that will cause greater ventilation relative to perfusion. Alveolar septal degeneration occurs in individuals with emphysema. The loss of alveolar surface area decreases gas exchange across the alveolar capillary membrane, which increases deadspace. Another cause of an elevated deadspace in emphysema is that pulmonary capillary destruction accompanies the alveolar septal degeneration. This also creates ventilation in excess of perfusion. Positive pressure ventilation preferentially delivers more of the gas volume to nongravity-dependent areas of the lung without a change in cardiac output. Those lung areas receive ventilation in excess of perfusion and become deadspace units. Additionally, positive pressure ventilation dilates the airways during inspiration, which also slightly increases anatomic deadspace.

Shunt-producing pathology can be classified into three types: anatomic, capillary and perfusion in excess of ventilation. Shapiro identifies different pathologic or clinical conditions that could cause each of the above types of shunt.

Anatomic shunt increases if the individual has a greater volume of venous blood returning to left heart without circulating through the lung. *Congenital heart disease, pulmonary fistula* or *vascular lung tumors* are types of problems that increase anatomic shunt and may seriously impair oxygenation.

Capillary shunt may develop if lung pathology is abnormal. *Acute atelectasis, alveolar fluid* and *consolidation* are all clinical conditions that decrease the patient's oxygenation because alveoli are either collapsed and gas exchange is unable to occur or the alveoli are so filled with debris and/or fluid that they are unable to normally exchange oxygen. The blood flowing past these alveoli is not oxygenated and returns to the left heart as venous blood. The amount of capillary shunting present is directly proportional to the amount of alveolar surface area that is involved in the pathologic process.

Perfusion in excess of ventilation or low $\dot{V}/\dot{Q}$ is the last type of shunt-producing pathology. It is also known as shunt effect or venous admixture. *Hypoventilation, uneven distribution of ventilation* and *diffusion defect* are causes of this type of shunt. Hypoventilation and uneven distribution of ventilation result in global or localized areas of low $\dot{V}/\dot{Q}$. A diffusion defect may also cause hypoxemia. For example, an individual with pulmonary fibrosis may be hypoxemic at rest due to low $\dot{V}/\dot{Q}$. However, during exertion (walking), the individual's circulation time decreases (increased CO), and the diseased pulmonary parenchyma cannot saturate the hemoglobin in the reduced time it is in the pulmonary capillaries. Therefore, the individual cannot maintain resting P_aO_2 during exertion and hypoxemia worsens.

Deadspace and shunt are also discussed in Chapters 9 and 7 respectively of the text and the workbook. Please refer to them if a more extensive review is required.

The author presents patient cases to illustrate his discussion of shunt and deadspace. The examples allow the reader to understand how deadspace and shunt are manifested in the majority of clinical circumstances. Shapiro emphasizes that these cases are teaching tools and not all patients follow these clinical patterns. These are guidelines, NOT rules, and are intended to help clinicians understand the differences between shunt and deadspace in the majority of patients.

If the diagnosis is pulmonary embolism, the patient's clinical data may follow this pattern.

Deadspace-producing Pathology Case Example

A 60-year-old, 48-kg woman with a two-day history of deep venous thrombosis complains suddenly of chest pain and shortness of breath. She was breathing room air (F_IO_2 of 0.21). The following clinical information is available:

ABGs: pH 7.48, P_aCO_2 33 mmHg, P_aO_2 60 mmHg, F_IO_2 0.21
Vital signs: BP 140/70, P 110/min, T 37.8° C
PFT: V_T 600 ml, RR 25/min, $\dot{V}_E$ 15 L/min

The patient's acid-base condition indicates a slight hyperventilation with mild hypoxemia. The patient's increased minute volume is approximately three times normal with a P_aCO_2 only slightly less than normal (33 mmHg). This indicates increased deadspace ventilation.

The same patient was given oxygen therapy on a F_IO_2 of 0.50. After 20 minutes, the following clinical data is available:

ABGs: pH 7.45, P_aCO_2 35 mmHg, P_aO_2 110 mmHg, F_IO_2 0.5
Vital signs: BP 120/70, P 100/min, T 37.8° C
PFT: V_T 600 ml, RR 25/min, $\dot{V}_E$ 15 L/min

If a patient with increased deadspace ventilation is given oxygen therapy, cardiopulmonary work isn't significantly reduced despite the relief of the patient's hypoxemia. Increased deadspace necessitates a very inefficient breathing pattern. It requires that the individual double, triple or quadruple his/her $\dot{V}_E$ in order to maintain an adequate P_aCO_2. The additional respiratory muscle work consumes energy (increased VO_2) and requires greater blood flow, arterial oxygen content, nutritional substrates and ATP stores. Therefore, although administering oxygen to an individual with increased deadspace ventilation increases the P_aO_2, it doesn't reduce cardiopulmonary work significantly.

Shunt-producing Pathology Case Example

A 60-year-old, 48-kg woman with a two-day history of thrombophlebitis of the right calf complains suddenly of chest pain and shortness of breath. She was breathing room air (F_IO_2 of 0.21). The following clinical information is available:

ABGs: pH 7.52, P_aCO_2 27 mmHg, P_aO_2 60 mmHg, F_IO_2 0.21
Vital signs: BP 140/70, P 110/min, T 37.8° C
PFT: V_T 400 ml, RR 30/min, $\dot{V}_E$ 12 L/min

The patient's acid-base condition indicates acute hyperventilation with mild hypoxemia. The patient's increased minute volume is twice normal and consistent with the P_aCO_2 of 27 mmHg and a diagnosis of hyperventilation. The clinical data does not show a pattern that indicates an increase in deadspace.

The same patient was given oxygen therapy on a F_IO_2 of 0.50. After 20 minutes, the following clinical data is available:

ABGs: pH 7.48, P_aCO_2 33 mmHg, P_aO_2 90 mmHg, F_IO_2 0.5
Vital signs: BP 120/80, P 90/min, T 37.8° C
PFT: V_T 400 ml, RR 20/min, $\dot{V}_E$ 8 L/min

The patient's clinical data indicates that the response to oxygen is consistent with shunt-producing pathology (the patient is later found with a left lower lobe pneumonia). The cardiopulmonary work is reduced as evidenced by a reduction in the patient's $\dot{V}_E$, RR, P and BP. Oxygen therapy increases the P_AO_2 and subsequently the P_aO_2 in lung units with low $\dot{V}/\dot{Q}$ ratios. Therefore, the patient's hypoxemia is relieved and the compensatory cardiopulmonary response is reduced.

Key Points

- There are three major classifications of deadspace-producing pathology: anatomic deadspace, alveolar deadspace and ventilation in excess of perfusion.
- There are three major classifications of shunt-producing pathology: anatomic shunt, capillary shunt and perfusion in excess of ventilation.
- There are guidelines for distinguishing between deadspace-producing and shunt-producing pathologies.
- The redistribution of pulmonary perfusion secondary to decreased cardiac output or acute pulmonary hypertension increases the alveolar deadspace.
- Positive pressure ventilation or alveolar septal destruction may cause ventilation in excess of perfusion, which increases deadspace.
- Rapid, shallow breathing is the major cause of increased anatomic deadspace.
- Hypoventilation, uneven distribution of ventilation or diffusion defect may cause perfusion in excess of ventilation, which increases an individual's shunt effect.
- Acute atelectasis, alveolar edema or alveolar consolidation increases capillary shunting.
- Some types of congenital heart disease, pulmonary fistula or vascular lung tumors cause anatomic shunt.
- When cardiopulmonary reserves are adequate, hypertension and tachycardia are the clinical manifestations of increased cardiovascular work in cases of acute shunt or deadspace.
- Administering oxygen to individuals with acute deadspace-producing pathology has little effect on the individual's work of breathing or cardiovascular work.
- Oxygen therapy in individuals with shunt-producing pathology reduces the individual's cardiopulmonary work if a significant amount of venous admixture is present.

- In individuals with an acute increase in deadspace, the normal relationship between increased minute ventilation and decreased P_aCO_2 is not present (see Table 2).
- The guidelines for identifying patterns of response in individuals with shunt or deadspace won't be applicable in all patient situations. Remember: Some medical situations can be highly complex because of multiple superimposed problems. Central nervous system, metabolic, cardiovascular and pulmonary abnormalities (to name a few) complicate clinical situations so that the patient doesn't respond predictably.
- Alveolar PCO_2 is inversely proportional to alveolar ventilation and alveolar PO_2 is directly proportional to alveolar ventilation.
- Adequate cardiopulmonary reserves allow for compensatory changes in perfusion should ventilatory dysfunction occur and compensatory changes in ventilation should heart dysfunction occur. The purpose of these changes is to maintain homeostasis of the organism.

Formulas

Cardiac Output

$$CO = SV \times HR$$

Deadspace Ventilation

$$\dot{V}_D = \dot{V}_{Danat} + \dot{V}_{Dalv}$$

Minute Ventilation

$$\dot{V}_E = \dot{V}_A + \dot{V}_D \text{ or } MV = \dot{V}_A + \dot{V}_D$$

Physiologic Shunt Equation

$$\frac{\dot{Q}_{sp}}{\dot{Q}_T} = \frac{[C_cO_2 - C_aO_2]}{[C_cO_2 - C_{\bar{v}}O_2]}$$

Tables

Deadspace Producing	*Shunt Producing*
Anatomic 1. Rapid, shallow breathing	Anatomic 1. Congenital heart disease 2. Pulmonary fistula 3. Vascular lung tumors
Alveolar deadspace 1. Acute pulmonary embolus 2. Redistribute pulmonary perfusion a. Decreased cardiac output b. Acute pulmonary hypertension	Capillary shunting 1. Acute atelectasis 2. Alveolar fluid 3. Consolidation
Ventilation in excess of perfusion 1. Positive pressure ventilation 2. Alveolar septal destruction	Perfusion in excess of ventilation 1. Hypoventilation 2. Uneven distribution of ventilation 3. Diffusion defect

Table 1: Classification of deadspace and shunt-producing pathology.

MV(L)	*$\dot{V}_A$(L)*	*P_aCO_2 (mmHg)**
3	2	80
6	4	40
12	8	30
24	16	20

* The medical scientific community has recommended the use of International System of Units (SI), which calls for pressure to be expressed as kilopascals (kPa) rather than millimeters of mercury (mmHg). The conversion factor for mmHg to kPa is 0.133. Bicarbonate is expressed in millimoles per liter (mMol/L), which has a conversion factor of 1 with millequivalents per liter (mEq/L).

Table 2: Ideal minute ventilation, alveolar ventilation, and arterial carbon dioxide tension relationships.

	Deadspace-producing Pathology	***Shunt-producing Pathology***
$\dot{V}_E$	Increases not directly reflective of predicted P_aCO_2 (see Table 2)	Increases reflective of predicted P_aCO_2 (See Table 2)
ABG *	Normal or slightly decreased P_aCO_2 with accompanying hypoxemia	Acute alveolar hyperventilation with accompanying hypoxemia
CV work *	Increased as evidenced by hypertension and tachycardia	Increased as evidenced by hypertension and tachycardia
Effect of O_2	Significant increase in P_aO_2	** Significantly improved P_aO_2 after reduction of CP work
	Little or no change in P_aCO_2	** Increase in P_aCO_2 toward normal
	Little or no change in WOB as reflected in RR, use of accessory muscles or dyspnea	** Decreased WOB as reflected in decreased RR, use of accessory muscles, subjective relief of dyspnea
	Little change in CV work as reflected in BP and HR	** Decreased CV work as reflected in decreased BP and HR

* When cardiopulmonary reserves are adequate to meet the demands
** Assuming a significant element of venous admixture (low $\dot{V}/\dot{Q}$)

Table 3: Cardiopulmonary guidelines for pathologic conditions.

Problems

Select and mark the best answer.

1. Identify the categories of deadspace-producing and shunt-producing pathologies listed below.
   Key: **D** = deadspace category
   S = shunt category
   B = both categories

   _____ a. Alveolar
   _____ b. Anatomic
   _____ c. Capillary
   _____ d. Ventilation in excess of perfusion
   _____ e. Perfusion in excess of ventilation

2. Classify each of the diseases/conditions listed below according to whether it causes an increase in deadspace or an increase in shunt.
   Key: **D** = disorder that increases deadspace
   S = disorder that increases shunt

   _____ a. Hypoventilation
   _____ b. Rapid, shallow breathing
   _____ c. Decreased cardiac output
   _____ d. Congenital heart disease
   _____ e. Acute pulmonary embolism
   _____ f. Positive pressure ventilation
   _____ g. Pulmonary atelectasis
   _____ h. Alveolar fluid

3. Compare the effect oxygen therapy has on individuals with shunt-producing pathology with the effect it has on those with deadspace-producing pathology.

4. Define the following terms:

   a. Intrapulmonary shunt ____________________

   b. Deadspace ventilation ____________________

5. Classify each of the diseases/conditions listed below into the correct category of deadspace or shunt:

   a. Hypoventilation ____________________

   b. Rapid, shallow breathing ____________________

   c. Decreased cardiac output ____________________

   d. Congenital heart disease ____________________

   e. Acute pulmonary embolism ____________________

   f. Alveolar septal destruction ____________________

   g. Pulmonary atelectasis ____________________

   h. Alveolar fluid ____________________

   i. Acute pulmonary hypertension ____________________

6. If a patient has adequate cardiopulmonary reserve, what blood gas alterations are classically seen with shunt-producing pathology? (More than one answer may be correct.)
   a. The P_aCO_2 is normal or slightly decreased.
   b. The blood gas values show acute alveolar hyperventilation.
   c. The P_aCO_2 is elevated.
   d. The patient shows hypoxemia.
   e. Hypoxemia is not present.

7. What minute volume changes are seen in patients with shunt-producing pathology?
   a. Minute volume increases but does it not result in the predictable P_aCO_2 reduction.
   b. Minute volume does not change.
   c. Minute volume decreases with a predictable increase in the patient's P_aCO_2.
   d. Minute volume increases and directly correlates with the decrease in P_aCO_2.

8. If a patient has adequate cardiopulmonary reserve, what blood gas alterations are classically seen with deadspace-producing pathology? (More than one answer may be correct.)
   a. The P_aCO_2 is normal or slightly decreased.
   b. The blood gas values show acute alveolar hyperventilation.
   c. The P_aCO_2 is elevated.
   d. The patient shows hypoxemia.
   e. Hypoxemia is not present.

A 65-year-old male with a seven-year history of congestive heart failure was admitted because of a worsening of his shortness of breath. He had the "flu" last week and had not recovered. His clinical data revealed the following information:

ABGs: pH 7.55, P_aCO_2 25 mmHg, P_aO_2 51 mmHg
Vital signs: BP 145/95, P 110/min
PFT: V_T 450 ml, RR 33/min, $\dot{V}_E$ 15 L

The patient was put on an F_IO_2 of 0.5, and after 20 minutes, his clinical signs and laboratory values showed the following changes:

ABGs: pH 7.50, P_aCO_2 30 mmHg, P_aO_2 75 mmHg
Vital signs: BP 135/90, P 96/min
PFT: V_T 450 ml, RR 23/min, $\dot{V}_E$ 10.3 L

Use this information to answer questions 9 and 10.

9. What is the probable cause of the patient's hypoxemia?

____

10. What is the patient's response to oxygen therapy in the following areas?

 a. P_aO_2 and P_aCO_2 response ____________________

 b. Work of breathing ____________________

 c. Cardiovascular work ____________________

Answers to Problems

1. a. D b. B c. S d. D e. S
 Items a, b, d are categories of deadspace-producing pathology. Items b, c, e are categories of shunt-producing pathology.

2. a. S b. D c. D d. S e. D f. D g. S h. S
 Items b, c, e, f are diseases/conditions that cause an increase in $\dot{V}_D$. Items a, d, g, h are diseases/conditions that cause an increase in $\dot{Q}_{sp}/\dot{Q}_T$.

3. The effects of supplemental oxygen are very different in patients with acute increases in deadspace compared with the effects in those with intrapulmonary shunt.

 P_aO_2 - The P_aO_2 in both clinical problems will increase in response to oxygen. The difference is that in shunt the increased P_aO_2 will occur only when cardiopulmonary work is reduced.

 P_aCO_2 - There are significant differences in the patients' P_aCO_2. In high deadspace, the P_aCO_2 will change very little in response to oxygen; but in shunt, the P_aCO_2 will increase toward normal because hypoxemia is relieved.

 WOB - Again, when comparing how the WOB is affected by the administration of oxygen, there are significant differences between the two patients. In high deadspace, work of breathing is not significantly relieved because of the high ventilatory work the patient must maintain. Increasing the P_aO_2 will not reduce WOB, but it will help the patient sustain it. In high shunt, the work of breathing decreases because hypoxemia is relieved. The hypoxemia is the underlying reason for the subjective feeling of breathlessness, use of accessory muscles, increased minute ventilation and respiratory rate. With the increase in P_aO_2, the WOB is reduced.

 CV work - The differences between CV responses in patients with deadspace and patients with shunt are similar to those seen in the work of breathing. In high deadspace, there is little change in CV work. The blood pressure and heart rate remain high because the patient's ventilatory work is still increased. In high shunt, the blood pressure and heart rate decrease because with the increase in P_aO_2, the compensatory cardiac response is reduced.

4. a. Intrapulmonary shunt - The portion of the cardiac output entering the left side of the heart that does not have perfect gas exchange with perfect alveoli. This is the definition of true shunt. Clinically, the physiologic shunt is a measurement of true shunt (anatomic and capillary) and venous admixture. Therefore, many patients with a physiologic shunt will respond to oxygen therapy to a limited degree. Their response is directly proportional to how much venous admixture is present. The greater the number of low $\dot{V}/\dot{Q}$ lung units, the more the patient will respond to oxygen.

 b. Deadspace ventilation - The volume of inspired air which does not take part in gas exchange. When the patient has an increase in deadspace, he/she must increase ventilation to maintain a normal P_aCO_2. This is a very inefficient breathing pattern and requires increased energy expenditure by the patient's respiratory muscles to sustain the high $\dot{V}_E$. If the condition persists, respiratory muscle fatigue develops and ventilation decreases, with eventual ventilatory failure.

5. a. Shunt-producing, perfusion in excess of ventilation
 b. Deadspace-producing, anatomic deadspace
 c. Deadspace-producing, alveolar deadspace
 d. Shunt-producing, anatomic shunt
 e. Deadspace-producing, alveolar deadspace
 f. Deadspace-producing, ventilation in excess of perfusion
 g. Shunt-producing, capillary shunt
 h. Shunt-producing, capillary shunt
 i. Deadspace-producing, alveolar deadspace

6. b, d: In shunt-producing pathology, the patients usually show acute alveolar hyperventilation with hypoxemia.

7. d: In shunt-producing pathology, the patient's minute volume increases with a proportional lowering of the P_aCO_2. The proportional relationship is not consistent with increased deadspace.

8. a, d: In deadspace-producing pathology, the patient's minute volume increases but the P_aCO_2 shows a normal or slightly reduced value. This is not a proportional relationship and indicates deadspace. The patient also has an accompanying hypoxemia.

9. Shunt-producing pathology

10. a. P_aO_2 and P_aCO_2 response: The patient's P_aO_2 increased, alleviating the hypoxemia. The patient's P_aCO_2 increased by 5 mmHg toward the normal range of 35-45 mmHg.
 b. Work of breathing: The patient's WOB decreased. The minute volume and respiratory rate decreased without a

change in tidal volume.
c. Cardiovascular work: The patient's cardiovascular work also decreased. The blood pressure decreased, as well as the heart rate.

Case Study

This 69-year-old white male was admitted through the emergency room with a four-hour history of severe chest pain, dyspnea, diaphoresis and nausea. He was discharged from the hospital one month ago.

Past Medical History:
One admission this year for CHF
Coronary artery bypass graft three years ago
Hypertension

Family History:
+ Heart disease
+ Hypertension

Social History:
Married, 4 children
60 pack/year smoking history

Physical Exam:
Oriented white male in acute distress.

Vital signs: BP = 160/90
HR = 110
RR = 36
T = 37.4° C

Height 5'8", Weight 65 kg
Chest: Prominent inspiratory crackles and coarse breath sounds auscultated throughout the chest

Cardiovascular: Elevated ST segments and Q waves present in V_2 and V_3 with a loss of voltage in the anterior leads. Atrial fibrillation present. Consistent with anterior MI.

Impression: Acute myocardial infarction
Pulmonary edema
COPD

Lab studies: WBC 8.2/mm^3, Na 127 mEq/L, K 6.0 mEq/L, Cl 92 mEq/L, Glucose 240 mg/dL, Hb/Hct WNL, Blood gas results on RA: pH 7.44, P_aCO_2 36, PO_2 51

Pulmonary Function: $\dot{V}_E$ 12 L, RR 30, V_T 400 ml

Day 1: The patient was admitted for chest pain and shortness of breath. At the time of admission, he was on diuretics, inotropic agents and antihypertensives. He was started on 0.40 F_IO_2.

Blood gas results on a F_IO_2 0.4: pH 7.42, P_aCO_2 38, PO_2 70
Pulmonary Function: $\dot{V}_E$ 12 L, RR 30, V_T 400 ml

Vital signs: BP = 147/90
Pulse = 100/min

1. Does this patient have primarily a shunt-producing problem or a deadspace-producing problem? Explain your answer.
2. What specific problem of shunt or deadspace does this patient have?
3. What problem or problems does the patient have that could cause the opposite condition from that which you identified in question 1?
4. Do you think this patient has adequate cardiopulmonary reserve? Explain your answer.
5. Discuss the possible causes and possible clinical problems associated with the patient's abnormal blood chemistry values.

Suggested Additional Readings

Kacmarek, RM, Mack, CW and Dimas, S, *The Essentials of Respiratory Care,* 3rd edition, C.V. Mosby, St. Louis, MO, 1990, Chapters 4 and 13 and pp. 406-410.

Pierson, DJ and Kacmarek, RM, *Foundations of Respiratory Care,* Churchill Livingstone, New York, NY, 1992, Chapters 10, 24, 26, 30 and 31.

Scanlan, CL, Spearman, CB and Sheldon, RL, *Egan's Fundamentals of Respiratory Care*, 5th edition, C.V. Mosby, St. Louis, MO, 1990, pp. 197-202, 606-608.

REVIEW QUESTIONS

Please pick the best answer for each question. Note that the number in parentheses indicates the chapter from which the question is taken.

1. Which statement correctly describes the normal distribution of ventilation in the lung? (2)
   a. Ventilation is the greatest in the dependent areas of the lung.
   b. Ventilation is the greatest in the anterior sections of the lung.
   c. Ventilation is the greatest in the upper lung zones.
   d. With normal airway resistance, ventilation is equal throughout the lung.

2. Which of the following is not a measure of central tendency? (5)
   a. Median
   b. Mode
   c. Arithmetic mean
   d. Standard deviation
   e. Both a and b are correct.

3. Which of the following statements is/are true with regard to decreased plasma HCO_3^- resulting in metabolic acidosis? (1)
   I. Tubular fluid bicarbonate has increased.
   II. Phosphate buffers are used to ↑ H^+ excretion.
   III. Ammonia buffers attempt to ↑ H^+ excretion.
   IV. pH will not change in these cases.

   a. I only
   b. I and IV
   c. II and IV
   d. II and V
   e. II and III

4. When P_aCO_2 increases by 20 mmHg, you would expect pH to change by _____ pH units. (5)
   a. +0.20
   b. –0.20
   c. +0.10
   d. –0.10
   e. There would be no change.

5. All else being unchanged, what is the effect of increasing a patient's Hb (gm/dL) on O_2 saturation? (4)
   a. Increases
   b. Decreases
   c. Remains unchanged
   d. The effect cannot be determined
   e. Both b and c are correct.

6. If the patient's mixed venous CO_2 content decreases with no change in alveolar ventilation or alveolar perfusion, what is the effect on alveolar CO_2? (3)
   a. Increases
   b. Decreases
   c. No change

7. Respiratory failure (6)
   a. includes ventilatory failure.
   b. includes oxygenation failure.
   c. does not include ventilatory failure.
   d. does not include oxygenation failure.
   e. Both a and b are correct.

8. Anion gap may be determined including or not including K^+ values in the calculations. What is the normal range for anion gap if we exclude the potassium concentration? (1)
   a. 6-10 mMol/L
   b. 14-20 mMol/L
   c. 8-14 gm%
   d. 10-12 gm%
   e. 8-16 mMol/L

9. If we include the $[K^+]$ values in our calculations of anion gap, what effect will that have on the anion gap normal range compared with the answer in question 8? (1)
   a. No change will occur.
   b. Direction of change cannot be determined.
   c. Anion gap values will increase.
   d. Anion gap values will decrease.
   e. K^+ should never be included in the calculation.

10. Jane Smith is a 62-year-old white female who has normal pulmonary functions. What do you estimate her P_aO_2 to be? (5)
    a. 96
    b. 78
    c. 72
    d. 68
    e. 87

11. "Buffering capacity" refers to the ability of a system to (1)
    a. withstand rapid and wide changes in physiologic pressure.
    b. moderate the effects of strong acids and strong bases.
    c. reduce the effects of transtissue fluid imbalances.
    d. produce large outcome effects from small input changes.
    e. increase the sensitivity of neuroregulatory receptors.

12. At standard conditions 1 liter of oxygen gas weighs approximately 1.44 grams and 1 liter of carbon dioxide weighs 1.98 grams. If you inject these two gases into a vacuum, which gas diffuses faster? (This is not in a liquid; therefore, don't consider solubility.) (2)
    a. Oxygen
    b. Carbon dioxide

13. How much faster does the gas diffuse that you identified in question 12? (2)
    a. 2 times faster
    b. 1.5 times faster
    c. 1.37 times faster
    d. 1.17 times faster

14. Classify each of the diseases/conditions listed below into the correct category of deadspace or shunt. (10)

    a. Pulmonary fistula
    ____
    b. Rapid, shallow breathing
    ____
    c. Decreased cardiac output
    ____
    d. Diffusion defect
    ____
    e. Pulmonary vascular tumor
    ____
    f. Alveolar septal destruction
    ____
    g. Pulmonary consolidation
    ____
    h. Uneven distribution of ventilation
    ____
    i. Acute pulmonary hypertension
    ____

15. CO has _____ the affinity for hemoglobin than does O_2. (4)
    a. one-third
    b. 25% of
    c. 10 times
    d. one-half
    e. 200-250 times

16. How is most of the carbon dioxide transported from the tissues to the lungs? (3)
    a. Chemical combination with hemoglobin
    b. Physically dissolved in the plasma
    c. As carbamino compounds in the plasma
    d. As bicarbonate ion

17. The normal hemoglobin content is (6)
    a. < 12 gm/dL.
    b. > 12 gm/dL.
    c. < 10 gm/dL.
    d. > 10 gm/dL.
    e. < 8 gm/dL.

18. With respect to work of breathing (WOB) (6)
    a. WOB increases as the day progresses.
    b. WOB decreases as energy stores decrease.
    c. increased WOB has a beneficial effect on pulmonary perfusion.
    d. WOB includes both internal respiration and external respiration.
    e. WOB causes respiratory distress.

Use the following information to answer questions 19-23.

Ima Smoker was on a spontaneous breathing trial with the goal of removal from mechanical ventilation and extubation. Her vital signs after 10 minutes on a tube trial were RR 32, BP 150/90, T 38° C, HR 110. Her ideal body weight was 50 kg. The respiratory care practitioner obtained the following pulmonary function measurements: Spontaneous V_T 300 ml, $\dot{V}_E$ 9.6 L, VC 500 ml, PIP –45 cm H_2O. Her ABGs were pH 7.55, P_aCO_2 25, P_aO_2 80, HCO_3^- 24, BE 0, S_aO_2 .98 on an F_IO_2 .4.

19. What is this patient's anatomic deadspace? (3)
    a. 30 cc/breath
    b. 50 cc/breath
    c. 110 cc/breath
    d. 150 cc/breath

20. What is this patient's alveolar ventilation? (3)
    a. 8.64 L
    b. 8.00 L
    c. 6.08 L
    d. 4.80 L

21. How would you classify this patient's respiratory acid-base status? (3)
    a. Compensated respiratory acidosis
    b. Uncompensated respiratory alkalosis
    c. Uncompensated respiratory acidosis
    d. Partially compensated respiratory alkalosis

22. If this patient's alveolar ventilation decreased, what would be the effect on her P_aCO_2? (3)
    a. It would not affect her P_aCO_2.
    b. It would decrease her P_aCO_2.
    c. It would increase her P_aCO_2.

23. If this patient's respiratory rate were 40 instead of 32, what would be the effect on her deadspace ventilation? (3)
    a. Deadspace ventilation would not change because anatomic deadspace is fixed.
    b. Deadspace ventilation would decrease because the lower respiratory rate decreases the total contribution $\dot{V}_D$ makes to the $\dot{V}_E$.
    c. Deadspace ventilation would increase because the higher respiratory rate increases the total contribution $\dot{V}_D$ makes to the $\dot{V}_E$.
    d. $\dot{V}_D$ would increase because it has an inverse relationship with respiratory rate.

24. Regarding P_aCO_2, which of the following is true? (9)
    a. All of the below are true.
    b. P_aCO_2 approximates P_ACO_2.
    c. P_aCO_2 is a qualitative index of $\dot{V}_A$.
    d. P_aCO_2 is not quantitative index of $\dot{V}_A$.
    e. P_aCO_2 is easier to assess than P_ACO_2.

25. Which of the following indicates the normal range for $\dot{V}_D/V_T$ in spontaneously breathing subjects? (9)
    a. 0.4-0.5
    b. 0.5-0.7
    c. 0.1-0.3
    d. 0.2-0.4
    e. 0.6-0.8

26. Which of the following arterial blood gases is consistent with uncompensated respiratory acidosis? (3)
    a. pH 7.28, P_aCO_2 76, HCO_3^- 35, BE +3.7
    b. pH 6.94, P_aCO_2 132, HCO_3^- 25, BE 0
    c. pH 7.36, P_aCO_2 69, HCO_3^- 38, BE +7
    d. pH 7.46, P_aCO_2 33, HCO_3^- 23, BE 0

27. The major difference between the ideal inspired PO_2 and the P_AO_2 is (4)
    a. water vapor pressure.
    b. nitrogen concentration.
    c. carbon dioxide pressure.
    d. Both a and c are correct.
    e. Both a and b are correct.

28. P_aCO_2 42 mmHg and pH 7.32 indicate (6)
    a. acute alveolar hyperventilation.
    b. subacute alveolar hyperventilation.
    c. partially compensated metabolic acidosis.
    d. metabolic alkalosis.
    e. metabolic acidosis.

29. Given the following data, calculate the $C_{(a-v)}O_2$: (8)

	Radial Artery	Pulmonary Artery
pH	7.39	7.46
PCO_2	45 mmHg	50 mmHg
PO_2	84 mmHg	76 mmHg
O_2 content	18 ml/dL	12 ml/dL

    a. 26 mmHg
    b. 5 gm%
    c. 8 mmHg
    d. 6 ml/dL
    e. 16 vol%

30. If alveolar perfusion increases with no change in alveolar ventilation and mixed venous CO_2 content, what is the effect on alveolar CO_2? (3)
    a. Increases
    b. Decreases
    c. No change
    d. The effect cannot be determined.

31. Given the following data, calculate the base excess/deficit: (5) pH observed = 7.25; P_aCO_2 = 60 mmHg; pH predicted = 7.30.

    a. +5 mMol/L
    b. –7.5 mMol/L
    c. –3.3 mMol/L
    d. –10 mMol/L
    e. +2.7 mMol/L

32. O_2 sat is derived by which formula? (4)
    a. $PO_2 - P_aCO_2$
    b. Actual HbO/Potential HbO
    c. $C_CO_2 \times 1.46$/RR
    d. ($\dot{Q}_T \times V_T$)/stroke volume
    e. $PCO_2 \times$ pH + PO_2

Match the statement or definition below to the most correct term. (7)

33. _____ True shunt
34. _____ Venous admixture
35. _____ Anatomic shunt
36. _____ Physiologic shunt
37. _____ Estimated shunt

a. An alternative method of measuring intrapulmonary shunt in those patients who do not have a pulmonary artery catheter in place and have adequate cardiovascular reserve.
b. Pathologic conditions such as tetralogy of fallot or tricuspid atresia will increase this type of shunt.
c. The shunt that occurs in any individual with a disease or condition that impairs the oxygen exchange across the alveolar capillary membrane.
d. The product of the sum of the individual's anatomic shunt and capillary shunt.
e. The shunt that is measured when the individual is receiving less than 100% inspired oxygen.
f. The oxygenation defect that occurs when blood comes in contact with alveolar units that have reduced ventilation.

38. Which of the following may be responsible for an increased anion gap? (1)
    a. Increased lactic acid
    b. Polymyxin-B IV drip
    c. Decreased magnesium
    d. Hyperbilirubinemia
    e. Decreased serum calcium

39. Which of the following situations will result in an acidotic condition in the blood? (1)
    a. ↓ H^+ in the blood, ↓ HCO_3^- elimination
    b. ↑ CO_2 content and proportional ↑ [HCO_3^-] of the blood

c. ↑ H^+ elimination from the cells, ↓ [HCO_3^-] in the blood
d. ↓ CO_2 content and proportional ↓ [HCO_3^-] of the blood
e. Changes in [CO_2], [HCO_3^-] and [H^+] in blood don't affect pH.

40. $C_{(a-v)}O_2$ is also known as (8)
a. oxygen utilization.
b. oxygen extraction.
c. oxygen saturation.
d. cardiac output.
e. cardiopulmonary ratio.

41. Assuming you are at the top of Mount Everest at an altitude of 29,141 feet, use Dalton's Law of Partial Pressures to calculate the partial pressure of oxygen (PO_2) at that altitude. (2)

P_B 244 mmHg	Trace Gases 0.7 mmHg
Nitrogen 193 mmHg	P_{H2O} 0.49 mmHg

a. 52.19 mmHg
b. 51 mmHg
c. 49.81 mmHg
d. 48.8 mmHg

42. Given a patient on controlled PPV, what would you expect the normal range of the $\dot{V}_D/V_T$ ratio to be? (9)
a. 0.4-0.6
b. 0.2-0.4
c. 0.3-0.7
d. 0.1-0.2
e. 0.8-1.0

43. Ketoacidosis is a common result of (1)
a. overeating.
b. kyphoscoliosis.
c. diabetes.
d. vegetarianism.
e. leukemia.

44. A common effect of PPV is (9)
a. Increased V_{Danat}.
b. Increased cardiac output.
c. Increased P_ECO_2.
d. Increased pulmonary perfusion.
e. Increased V_{Dalv}.

45. Variations from the central data point(s) are measured in terms of _____ from the middle of a symmetrical distribution. (5)
a. standard deviations
b. variance
c. modes
d. confidence levels
e. Both a and c are correct.

46. If cardiac output decreases after a myocardial infarction, what effect does this have on deadspace? (10)
a. Anatomic deadspace will increase.
b. Anatomic deadspace will decrease.
c. Alveolar deadspace will increase.
d. Alveolar deadspace will decrease.
e. There is no change in deadspace.

47. The most easily obtainable index of cellular oxygenation is (8)
a. P_aO_2.
b. S_aO_2.
c. $P_{(a-v)}O_2$.
d. $S_{(a-v)}O_2$.
e. $C_{(a-v)}O_2$.

48. $DO_2 - C_{(a-v)}O_2$ = (8)
a. S_aO_2.
b. $S_{\bar{v}}O_2$.
c. C_aO_2.
d. F_IO_2.
e. P_aO_2.

49. Given an initial pH of 7.40 and an initial P_aCO_2 of 40 mmHg, indicate the correct effects on HCO_3^- under conditions I and II.
I = P_aCO_2 ↑ 10 mmHg; II = P_aCO_2 ↓ 10 mmHg (5)

	I	II
a.	–1 mMol/L	+1 mMol/L
b.	+1 mMol/L	–2 mMol/L
c.	+2 mMol/L	–2 mMol/L
d.	–2 mMol/L	+1 mMol/L
e.	–1 mMol/L	+2 mMol/L

50. O_2 content (6)
a. includes bound O_2.
b. does not include bound O_2.
c. includes dissolved O_2.
d. does not include dissolved O_2.
e. Both a and c are correct.

51. The major limitation to the extravascular fluid (EVF) oxygen volume is (8)
a. arterial oxygenation tension.
b. S_pO_2.
c. $C_{(a-v)}O_2$.
d. venous capillary PO_2.
e. tissue to venous PCO_2 difference.

52. A quantity of neon exerts a pressure of 1400 mmHg at 25°C in a 500 ml container. What is the pressure of the neon at 50°C? (2)
a. 2345 mmHg
b. 1809 mmHg
c. 1517 mmHg
d. 1291 mmHg

53. What gas law is used to solve the problem in question 52? (2)
a. Boyle's Law
b. Henry's Law
c. Graham's Law
d. Charles' Law
e. Gay-Lussac's Law

54. Clinically significant hypoxemia occurs when P_aO_2 is less than (6)
a. 80 mmHg.
b. 75 mmHg.
c. 60 mmHg.
d. 40 mmHg.
e. 30 mmHg.

55. Henry's Law deals with (4)
a. diffusion.
b. membrane potential.
c. solubility.
d. gas density.
e. fractional pressures.

56. Given a measured oxygen content of 1.20 gm/dL, what is the percent saturation of the sample (to the nearest full %)? (4)
a. 90%
b. 95%
c. 85%
d. 80%
e. 100%

57. The major cause of hypoxemia secondary to acutely decreased cardiac output is (9)
a. increased P_ECO_2.
b. increased $(a–v)O_2$.
c. decreased $(a–v)O_2$.
d. decreased P_ECO_2.
e. increased V_T.

58. If $\dot{V}_D$ increases, to keep $\dot{V}_A$ constant (9)
a. $\dot{V}_E$ must increase.
b. $\dot{V}_E$ must decrease.
c. V_{Danat} must decrease.
d. V_{Dalv} must decrease.
e. Both c and d are correct.

59. Given a $\dot{Q}_T$ of 5 L/min and a $C_{(a-v)}O_2$ of 4.5 ml/dL, calculate the VO_2. (8)
a. 250 gm%
b. 150 ml/min
c. 225 ml/min
d. 200 ml/dL
e. 175 gm/dL

60. The term *internal respiration* refers to the exchange of oxygen and carbon dioxide between the (2)
a. heme portion of the hemoglobin molecule and the blood.
b. environment and the pulmonary capillary blood.
c. mitochrondria and the intracellular fluid.
d. systemic capillary blood and the cells.

61. What percent of the oxygen content of the blood is responsible for maintaining the P_aO_2? (4)
a. 1-3%
b. 5-10%
c. 20-40%
d. 50-60%
e. 80-90%

62. Which of the following contains a representative sample of mixed venous pulmonary capillary blood? (8)
a. Pulmonary artery
b. Right ventricle
c. Inferior vena cava
d. Left atrium
e. Superior vena cava

63. Given a % F_IO_2 of 60%, calculate the minimum acceptable P_aO_2. (5)
a. 109 mmHg
b. 150 mmHg
c. 200 mmHg
d. 235 mmHg
e. 300 mmHg

64. If the temperature of a beach ball containing 10 liters of gas is decreased from 40° C to 35° C, what will be the new volume in the beach ball? (2)
a. 8.75 liters
b. 9.84 liters
c. 9.64 liters
d. 10.16 liters

65. What gas law is used to solve the problem in question 64? (2)
a. Boyle's Law
b. Henry's Law
c. Graham's Law
d. Charles' Law
e. Gay-Lussac's Law

66. The normal A-a oxygen gradient is (5)
a. 4 mmHg.
b. 80 mmHg.
c. 101 mmHg.
d. 1 mmHg/year of age.
e. 0 mmHg.

67. Pulmonary perfusion in Zone 1 of the lung is (2)
a. increased.
b. normal.
c. minimal or absent.

68. Which tissues do not normally utilize anaerobic metabolism? (1)
    a. Cardiac muscle cells
    b. Brain cells
    c. Red blood cells
    d. White blood cells
    e. Skeletal muscle cells

69. P_aCO_2 34 mmHg and pH 7.46-7.50 indicate (6)
    a. acute alveolar hyperventilation.
    b. subacute alveolar hyperventilation.
    c. partially compensated metabolic acidosis.
    d. metabolic alkalosis.
    e. metabolic acidosis.

70. Increasing $\dot{Q}_T$ will (8)
    a. increase $C_{(a-v)}O_2$.
    b. decrease $C_{(a-v)}O_2$.
    c. increase C_aO_2.
    d. Both a and c are correct.
    e. Both b and c are correct.

71. Indicate the proper initial $NaHCO_3$ dose to correct a base deficit of 15 mMol/L in a 30-year-old male. (5)
    a. 7.5 mMol/L
    b. 10.0 mMol/L
    c. 12.5 mMol/L
    d. 15.0 mMol/L
    e. 17.5 mMol/L

72. Which of the following CO_2 transport mechanisms carries the lowest total volume of CO_2? (3)
    a. Dissolved in the plasma
    b. Carried as bicarbonate ion
    c. In chemical combination with the protein globin in the hemoglobin
    d. Carried in combination with other buffers, e.g., phosphates

73. Increased V_{Danat} (9)
    a. increases respiration.
    b. decreases respiration.
    c. has no effect on respiration.
    d. decreases ventilation.
    e. increases ventilation.

74. How many globin molecules are in a hemoglobin molecule? (4)
    a. 4
    b. 6
    c. 3
    d. 2
    e. 1

75. Match the mathematical expression formula to the physical law it describes. (2)

___ Graham's Law	a. $P = p_1 + p_2 + p_3 + \ldots$
___ Respiratory Exchange Ratio (RR)	b. $P_1V_1 = P_2V_2$
___ Boyle's Law	c. $\frac{V_1}{T_1} = \frac{V_2}{T_2}$
___ Dalton's Law of Partial Pressures	d. $\frac{r_1}{r_2} = \frac{d_2}{d_1}$
___ Gay-Lussac's Law	e. $\frac{\text{Volume } CO_2 \text{ excreted}}{\text{Volume } O_2 \text{ uptake}}$
___ Charles' Law	f. $\frac{P_1}{T_1} = \frac{P_2}{T_2}$
	g. $\frac{\text{Volume } CO_2 \text{ produced}}{\text{Volume } O_2 \text{ consumed}}$

76. Using the following clinical information, calculate the estimated shunt: (7)
    Hb 12 gm% BP 125/66 T 37° C
    Hct 36% HR 90 beats/min RR 15 bpm
    P_B 740 mmHg, P_{H_2O} 47 mmHg

    Blood gases on CMV, F_IO_2 0.4
    Arterial pH 7.50, PCO_2 30, PO_2 65, S_aO_2 95%

77. Which of the following indicates an inefficient oxygen extraction ratio given stable $\dot{Q}_T$? (8)
    I. Increased oxygen demand
    II. Decreased oxygen content
    III. Decreased hemoglobin concentration

    a. I, II and III
    b. I and III
    c. I and II
    d. II only
    e. II and III

78. P_aCO_2 32 mmHg and pH 7.33 suggest (6)
    a. acute alveolar hyperventilation.
    b. subacute alveolar hyperventilation.
    c. partially compensated metabolic acidosis.
    d. metabolic alkalosis.
    e. metabolic acidosis.

79. Hemoglobin (Hb) exists as a weak acid in the red cell because it is (1)
    a. in equilibrium with the weak K^+ salt KHb.
    b. the conjugate acid of a strong base FeHb3.
    c. an H^+ donor and a HCO_3^- receiver.

d. a regulator of the extracellular acidosis of K^+ depletion.
e. a substitute for the $[Cl^-]$ ion in the erythrocyte.

80. HbMet is caused by (4)
a. methyl alcohol ingestion.
b. reduced serum oxygen partial pressures due to hypoxemic shunting.
c. oxidation of ferrous ions into ferric ions in the hemoglobin.
d. addition of two gamma polypeptide chains to the heme molecule.
e. failure to reduce dissolved CO_2 levels in the venous circulation.

81. Which statement correctly describes the normal distribution of perfusion in the lungs? (2)
a. Perfusion is the greatest in the lower zone of the lung.
b. Perfusion is the greatest in the middle zone of the lung.
c. Perfusion is the greatest in the upper zone of the lung.
d. Perfusion is equal throughout all the zones of the lung.

82. Atelectasis is an example of what type of intrapulmonary shunt? (7)
a. Anatomic
b. Capillary
c. Estimated
d. Venous admixture

83. $P_aCO_2 < 35$ mmHg and pH > 7.45 denote (6)
a. acute alveolar hyperventilation.
b. subacute alveolar hyperventilation.
c. partially compensated metabolic acidosis.
d. metabolic alkalosis.
e. metabolic acidosis.

84. Identify by putting a check next to each parameter which is consistent with the physiologic changes that occur in a patient with partially compensated respiratory alkalosis. (3)
Key: ↑ increased, ↓ decreased, <—> remains the same)
a. P_aCO_2: ___ ↑ ___ ↓ ___ <—>
b. pH: ___ ↑ ___ ↓ ___ <—>
c. HCO_3^-: ___ ↑ ___ ↓ ___ <—>
d. Base Excess: ___ ↑ ___ ↓ ___ <—>

85. Which of the following statements is true concerning changes in pulmonary perfusion? (2)
a. The upper borders of the pulmonary perfusion Zones 2 and 3 move higher when cardiac output decreases.
b. The upper borders of the pulmonary perfusion Zones 2 and 3 move downward when cardiac output decreases.
c. Cardiac output does not affect the size of the three individual lung zones.

86. Using the following clinical information, calculate the physiologic shunt: (7)
Hb 10 gm% BP 100/66 T 37.1° C
Hct 30% HR 110 beats/min RR 20 bpm
P_B 740 mmHg, P_{H2O} 47 mmHg

Pulmonary artery values: PAP 45/30 mmHg
PCWP 22 mmHg, RAP 18 mmHg, CO 3.80 LPM

Blood gases on CMV, F_IO_2 0.6, PEEP 10
Arterial pH 7.53, PCO_2 30, PO_2 60, S_aO_2 92%
Mixed venous pH 7.46, PCO_2 36, PO_2 32, $S_{\bar{v}}O_2$ 60%

87. Given a % F_IO_2 of 40%, which of the following represents corrected hypoxemia? (6)
a. P_aO_2 75 mmHg
b. O_2 Sat 94%
c. P_aCO_2 44 mmHg
d. P_aO_2 120 mmHg
e. P_aCO_2 50 mmHg

88. Decreased oxyhemoglobin affinity is shown by (6)
a. increased S_aO_2 at a given value of P_aO_2.
b. increased oxygen content of the blood.
c. increased dissolved oxygen.
d. a left shift of the oxygen dissociation curve.
e. a right shift of the oxygen dissociation curve.

89. Standard bicarbonate is (1)
a. an estimate of CO_2 combining power at $PO_2 = 100$.
b. an example of an unreliable calculated value.
c. the difference between HCO_3^- content and HCO_3^- capacity.
d. the CO_2 content of blood at $PCO_2 = 40$ mmHg, T = 37°C.
e. a new term for "base deficit."

90. What criteria are consistent with acute respiratory acidosis? (3)
a. Elevated pH, low P_aCO_2, normal HCO_3^- and normal base excess
b. Elevated pH, low P_aCO_2, low HCO_3^- and low base excess
c. Low pH, high P_aCO_2, high HCO_3^- and high base excess
d. Low pH, high P_aCO_2, normal HCO_3^- and normal base excess

91. When a ferrous ion is bonded in a porphyrin ring to form the heme molecule, how many covalent bond sites are free to bond with oxygen? (4)
a. 6
b. 8
c. 1
d. 3
e. 5

92. If a patient has adequate cardiopulmonary reserve, what blood gas alteration is classically seen with deadspace-producing pathology? (More than one answer may be correct.) (10)
   a. The P_aCO_2 is normal or slightly decreased.
   b. The blood gas values show acute alveolar hyperventilation.
   c. The P_aCO_2 is elevated.
   d. The patient shows hypoxemia.
   e. Hypoxemia is not present.

93. A 70-kg patient with decreasing lung compliance secondary to pneumonia has the following clinical profile: (10) pH 7.50, PCO_2 30 mmHg, PaO_2 65 mmHg, $\dot{V}_E$ 12 L, RR 35. Which of the following statements concerning this patient is correct? (More than one answer may be correct.)
   a. The patient has an increase in alveolar deadspace.
   b. The patient has an increase in anatomic deadspace.
   c. The patient has a decrease in alveolar deadspace.
   d. The patient has an increase in capillary shunting.
   e. The patient has a decrease in anatomic shunting.

94. Increasing serum CO_2 results in all of the following except (1)
   a. increased PCO_2.
   b. decreased intercellular $[H^+]$.
   c. increased H^+ ion excretion.
   d. increased $[CO_2]$ in the renal tubules.
   e. increased $[HCO_3^-]$ in the blood.

95. Which of the following equations could be used to determine alveolar ventilation? (3)
   a. $\dot{V}_E - \dot{V}_D$
   b. $\dot{V}_E - \dot{V}_A$
   c. $RR \times V_T$
   d. $\dot{V}_A + \dot{V}_D$

96. In critically ill patients (8)
   a. changes in $C_{(a-v)}O_2$ precede changes in P_aO_2.
   b. changes in $C_{(a-v)}O_2$ lag behind changes in P_aO_2.
   c. changes in $C_{(a-v)}O_2$ cause changes in P_aO_2.
   d. changes in $C_{(a-v)}O_2$ are the result of changes in P_aO_2.
   e. changes in $C_{(a-v)}O_2$ are related only to changes in [Hb].

97. Which of the following best defines alveolar hyperventilation (V_{alv})? (6)
   a. $V_{alv} = V_{Dphys} - V_{Danat}$
   b. $V_{alv} = V_T + (V_{Dphys} - V_{Danat})$
   c. $V_{alv} = V_T - (V_{Dphys} - V_{Danat})$
   d. $V_{alv} = V_T - (V_{Dphys} + V_{Danat})$
   e. $V_{alv} = V_{Dphys} + V_{Danat}$

98. As MV increases, which of the following is least likely to change? (5)
   a. P_aCO_2
   b. V_T
   c. $\dot{V}_A$
   d. V_{Dphys}
   e. V_{Danat}

99. If P_aO_2 increases as indicated in conditions I and II, identify the effect on pH. Assume the following initial values: pH 7.40, P_aCO_2 40 mmHg.
   $I = P_aCO_2 \downarrow 10$ mmHg, $II = P_aCO_2 \uparrow 10$ mmHg (5)

	I	II
a.	+0.10 units	–0.10 units
b.	–0.05 units	+0.10 units
c.	+0.05 units	–0.10 units
d.	–0.10 units	+0.05 units
e.	+0.10 units	–0.05 units

100. Normal V_{Danat} equals (9)
   a. 1 ml/kg.
   b. 2.2 ml/kg.
   c. 2.2 ml/lb.
   d. 3 ml/lb.
   e. 3 ml/kg.

101. Normal oxygen content of adult human blood is (4)
   a. 6.28 gm/L.
   b. 150 mmHg.
   c. 20.1 ml/dL
   d. 47 Torr.
   e. 100 mgm%.

102. Place a check next to those physiologic variables that that are necessary in order to calculate the intrapulmonary shunt. (7)

_____ a. C_cO_2	_____ g. P_AO_2
_____ b. Kcal/min	_____ h. C_aO_2
_____ c. $P_{\bar{v}}O_2$	_____ i. Arterial pH
_____ d. P_aCO_2	_____ j. Barometric pressure
_____ e. $S_{\bar{v}}O_2$	_____ k. Hemoglobin
_____ f. Mixed venous pH	_____ l. Arterial BP

103. Acute decreases in cardiac output and acute pulmonary hypertension both cause increases in lung (9)
   a. Zone 3.
   b. Zone 1.
   c. Zone 2.
   d. Both a and b are correct.
   e. Both b and c are correct.

104. If a patient's physiologic shunt has a significant element of venous admixture, what is the effect of oxygen administration on the arterial blood gas values? (10) (More than one answer may be correct.)
   a. The P_aCO_2 increases toward the normal range.
   b. The blood gas values continue to show acute alveolar hyperventilation with no change in the P_aCO_2.
   c. The P_aCO_2 is elevated and the P_aO_2 increases toward normal.
   d. The patient shows refractory hypoxemia.

e. The P_aO_2 improves after cardiopulmonary work decreases.

105. Which of the following is not a common adult Hb variant? (4)
a. HbCO
b. HbO
c. HbMet
d. HbF
e. HbS

106. Given a normal DO_2 (1,000 ml/min) and a C_aO_2 of 18 ml/dL, calculate the projected cardiac output ($\dot{Q}_T$). (8)

107. MV to P_aCO_2 disparity means (9)
a. MV in ml/minute does not equal P_aCO_2 in mmHg.
b. increased MV does not result in proportional changes in P_ACO_2.
c. P_aCO_2 exceeds MV × 0.03 (respiratory rate) + patient age.
d. Both a and b are correct.
e. $(P_aO_2 - P_aCO_2) = MV/12$.

108. Respiratory acidosis is a sign of ventilatory failure. (6)
a. True.
b. True, if oxygenation is normal.
c. True, if oxygenation is abnormal.
d. False.
e. False, if HCO_3^- is elevated.

109. The physiologic solution to lactic acidosis is (1)
a. plasma calcium retention.
b. increased anaerobic metabolism.
c. plasma calcium retention.
d. restoration of aerobic metabolism.
e. polysaccharide inhibition.

110. Acceptable ranges for pH and P_aCO_2 are (6)
a. narrower (less) than the normal ranges.
b. equal to the normal ranges.
c. wider (bigger) than the normal ranges.
d. not used in critical care.
e. within a SD of the average values.

111. Increased blood transit time will _____ pulmonary capillary oxygenation. (4)
a. decrease
b. increase
c. not change
d. Both a and c are correct.
e. Both b and c are correct.

112. Increased pulmonary vascular resistance (PVR) such as that caused by acute pulmonary hypertension (APH) (9)
a. increases perfusion in Zones 1 and 2.
b. increases perfusion in Zones 2 and 3.
c. increases perfusion in Zones 1 and 3.
d. increases perfusion in Zone 1 only.
e. decreases perfusion in all zones.

113. A difference of 4 mmHg in a-A PCO_2 indicates (9)
a. increased CO_2 production.
b. decreased $\dot{V}_D$.
c. increased V_T.
d. increased $\dot{V}_D$.
e. normal variations in ventilation.

114. Areas of the lung known as zero $\dot{V}/\dot{Q}$ units are also known as (9)
a. bypass units.
b. collateral units.
c. deadspace units.
d. high compression units.
e. shunt units.

115. Which of the following is the formula of the estimated shunt equation? (7)

a. $\dfrac{\dot{Q}_S}{\dot{Q}_T} = \dfrac{[C_cO_2 - C_aO_2]}{[C_cO_2 - C_{\bar{v}}O_2]}$

b. $\dfrac{\dot{Q}_{sp}}{\dot{Q}_T} = \dfrac{[C_cO_2 - C_aO_2]}{[C_aO_2 - C_{\bar{v}}O_2] + [C_cO_2 - C_aO_2]}$

c. $\dfrac{\dot{Q}_{sp}}{\dot{Q}_T} = \dfrac{[C_cO_2 - C_aO_2]}{3.5 + [C_cO_2 - C_aO_2]}$

d. $\dfrac{\dot{Q}_{SP}}{\dot{Q}_T} = \dfrac{(\dot{Q}_T)([C_aO_2 - C_{\bar{v}}O_2])\ (10)}{3.5 + [C_cO_2 - C_aO_2]}$

116. Which of the following equations could be used to determine an individual's anatomic deadspace? (3)
a. 1 ml/kg of ideal body weight
b. 1 ml/lb of ideal body weight
c. $\dot{V}_E + \dot{V}_A$
d. RR × V_T

117. Identify by putting a check next to each parameter which is consistent with the physiologic changes that occur in a patient with uncompensated respiratory alkalosis. (3)
Key: ↑ increased, ↓ decreased, <—> remains the same
a. P_aCO_2: ___ ↑ ___ ↓ ___<—>
b. pH: ___ ↑ ___ ↓ ___<—>
c. HCO_3^-: ___ ↑ ___ ↓ ___<—>
d. Base Excess: ___ ↑ ___ ↓ ___<—>

118. Which of the following oxygen tension indices has the greatest correlation with the physiologic shunt equation? (7)
a. Respiratory index
b. Oxygenation ratio
c. Alveolar oxygen ratio
d. Alveolar-arterial oxygen gradient

119. What effect does pulmonary embolism have on deadspace or intrapulmonary shunting? (10)
a. It causes capillary shunting.

b. It increases alveolar deadspace.
c. It increases anatomic deadspace.
d. It causes perfusion in excess of ventilation.

120. The difference between the measured pH and the predicted respiratory pH is the (5)
a. metabolic pH.
b. P_aCO_2 value.
c. total CO_2.
d. P_ACO_2 value.
e. projected HCO_3^- value.

121. Adequate renal blood flow is necessary to maintain "normal" metabolic acid balance. (1)
a. True.
b. False.
c. True, as long as the renal epithelium cells produce carbonic anhydrase.
d. False, if the renal tubules retain H^+ ions.
e. Only if the renal tubules' blood has reduced PCO_2.

122. The MV - P_aCO_2 relationship closely approximates the ______ relationship. (9)
a. P_ECO_2 - P_aCO_2
b. F_ECO_2 -P_ACO_2
c. $\dot{V}_A$ - P_aCO_2
d. V_{Danat} - P_aCO_2
e. VO_2 - F_IO_2

123. What effect would one expect to see if an increase in [Hb] resulted in 7% of the Hb being unsaturated? (4)
a. If the 7% was more than 5 gm/dL, Hb cyanosis would occur.
b. The SO_2 would increase by the change in Hb times 1.34.
c. PCO_2 would rise in response to the Haldane effect.
d. Hematocrit would fall proportionally to the increased Hb.
e. There would be no effect with such a small Hb change.

124. What minute volume changes are seen in patients with deadspace-producing pathology? (10)
a. Minute volume increases but it does not result in the predictable P_aCO_2 reduction.
b. Minute volume does not change.
c. Minute volume decreases with a predictable increase in the patient's P_aCO_2.
d. Minute volume increases and directly correlates with the decrease in P_aCO_2.

125. About _____% of the oxygen in the blood is in the bound state. (4)
a. 27
b. 33
c. 59
d. 75
e. 98

126. Which of the following acids is an important part of the acid-base mechanism? (1)
a. Keto
b. Lactic
c. Carbonic
d. Hydrochloric
e. Acetic

127. An acute change in P_aCO_2 from 40 mmHg to 50 mmHg should result in a pH change from 7.40 to (5)
a. 7.45.
b. 7.50.
c. 7.30.
d. 7.35.
e. 7.42.

128. Which of the following is an antioxidant mechanism? (8)
a. High hemoglobin concentration
b. Low carbon dioxide concentration
c. High nitrogen concentration
d. Cytrochrome dioxigenase concentration
e. Increased cardiac output

129. Areas of the lung known as infinite $\dot{V}/\dot{Q}$ units are also called (9)
a. bypass units.
b. collateral units.
c. low compression units.
d. deadspace units.
e. shunt units.

130. Nonanion gap acidosis may occur under which condition? (1)
a. Vomiting
b. Constipation
c. Urine retention
d. Sarcoidosis
e. Polymorphocytosis

131. Arterial oxygen tension is (6)
a. measured as P_aO_2.
b. the partial pressure of oxygen in arterial blood.
c. an example of Dalton's Law.
d. accurate between 30 and 200 mmHg.
e. All of the above are correct.

132. Which of the following statements is true concerning the end-pulmonary capillary oxygen content (C_CO_2)? (More than one answer may be correct.) (7)
a. It represents the function of the ideal lung.
b. Its value is less than arterial oxygen content.
c. The ideal alveolar gas equation is used to help determine the end-pulmonary capillary oxygen content.
d. It is used in the Fick equation for determining oxygen consumption.

133. What effect does pulmonary atelectasis have on deadspace or intrapulmonary shunt? (10)

a. It causes capillary shunting.
b. It increases alveolar deadspace.
c. It increases anatomic deadspace.
d. It increases anatomic shunting.

134. Which of the following categories of tissue hypoxia is associated with decreased oxygen carrying ability in the blood? (2)
a. Anemic hypoxia
b. Hypoxemic hypoxia
c. Histotoxic hypoxia
d. Circulatory hypoxia

135. Given the following information, calculate the $\dot{V}_D/V_T$ ratio and indicate the "normality" of the ratio for a healthy individual:
P_aCO_2 44 mmHg, P_ECO_2 33 mmHg. (9)
a. 0.25 abnormal
b. 0.25 normal
c. 0.30 normal
d. 0.30 abnormal
e. The ratio cannot be calculated with the data given.

136. P_{50} is (4)
a. the partial pressure increase caused by adding 50 molecules of oxygen to 100 ml of blood.
b. the point on the oxyhemoglobin curve where P_aCO_2 and P_aO_2 are each at 50% of their normal values.
c. the minute volume which will reduce a P_aCO_2 by half.
d. the P_aO_2 at which blood is 50% saturated at BTPS and a P_aCO_2 of 40 mmHg.
e. the metabolic rate which will utilize 50% of the oxygen stores in the body.

137. Base excess/deficit tells us the body's ability to (5)
a. produce $NaHCO_3$.
b. reduce Na^+ pump transport.
c. moderate the effect of $[H^+]$ changes.
d. change the rate CO_2 elimination.
e. change the amount of urine output.

138. Which of the following describes a "silent" lung unit? (2)
a. A unit of the lung that is neither ventilated nor perfused
b. A unit of the lung that is ventilated but not perfused
c. A unit of the lung that is perfused but not ventilated
d. A unit of the lung that has equal ventilation and perfusion

139. Which of the following best describes the term *normal range*? (5)
a. Median +/– 2 units
b. Mean +/– 2 SD
c. Mode +/– mean
d. Symmetrical range
e. Bell curve

140. $C_{(a-v)}O_2$ is affected by (8)
a. amount of deoxygenated venous admixture.
b. carbon dioxide production.
c. site of vascular catheter tip.
d. metabolic oxygen use.
e. a, c and d are correct.

Answers to Review Questions

1. a
2. d
3. e
4. d
5. c
6. b
7. e
8. e
9. c
10. b
11. b
12. a
13. d
14. a. anatomic shunt
    b. anatomic deadspace
    c. alveolar deadspace
    d. perfusion in excess of ventilation
    e. anatomic shunt
    f. ventilation in excess of perfusion
    g. capillary shunt
    h. perfusion in excess of ventilation
    i. alveolar deadspace
15. e
16. d
17. b
18. c
19. c
20. c
21. b
22. c
23. c
24. a
25. d
26. b
27. d
28. e
29. d
30. a
31. c
32. b
33. d
34. f
35. b
36. e
37. a
38. a
39. c
40. b
41. c
42. a
43. c
44. e
45. a
46. c
47. e
48. b
49. b
50. e
51. d
52. c
53. e
54. c
55. c
56. a
57. c
58. a
59. c
60. d
61. a
62. a
63. e
64. b
65. d
66. a
67. c
68. a
69. b
70. e
71. a
72. a
73. c
74. e
75. d, e, b, a, f, c
76. 27%

Estimated Shunt Equation:

$$\frac{\dot{Q}_{sp}}{\dot{Q}_T} = \frac{[C_{C}O_2 - C_aO_2]}{3.5 + [C_{C}O_2 - C_aO_2]}$$

$C_{C}O_2 = 1.00\,(12 \times 1.34) + (240\text{ mmHg} \times 0.0031)$
$16.82\text{ ml/dL} = 16.08\text{ ml/dL} + 0.743\text{ ml/dL}$
$C_aO_2 = .95(12 \times 1.34) + (75\text{ mmHg} \times 0.0031)$
$15.51\text{ ml/dL} = 15.28\text{ ml/dL} + 0.232\text{ ml/dL}$

With the above information, the $\frac{\dot{Q}_{sp}}{\dot{Q}_T}$ can now be calculated:

$$\frac{\dot{Q}_{sp}}{\dot{Q}_T} = \frac{16.82\,^{ml}/_{dL} - 15.51\,^{ml}/_{dL}}{3.5 + [16.82\,^{ml}/_{dL} - 15.51\,^{ml}/_{dL}]}$$

$$= \frac{1.31\,^{ml}/_{dL}}{3.5\,^{ml}/_{dL} + 1.31\,^{ml}/_{dL}}$$

$$= \frac{1.31\,^{ml}/_{dL}}{4.81\,^{ml}/_{dL}} \times 100$$

$$\frac{\dot{Q}_{sp}}{\dot{Q}_T} = 27\%$$

77. a
78. c
79. a
80. c
81. a
82. b
83. a
84. a. ↓
    b. ↑
    c. ↓
    d. ↓
85. b
86. 32%

Physiologic Shunt Equation:

$$\frac{\dot{Q}_{sp}}{\dot{Q}_T} = \frac{[C_cO_2 - C_aO_2]}{[C_cO_2 - C_{\bar{v}}O_2]}$$

$C_cO_2 = 1.00\,(10 \times 1.34) + (378 \text{ mmHg} \times 0.0031)$
$14.57 \text{ ml/dL} = 13.4 \text{ ml/dL} + 1.173 \text{ ml/dL}$
$C_aO_2 = .92(10 \times 1.34) + (60 \text{ mmHg} \times 0.0031)$
$12.52 \text{ ml/dL} = 12.33 \text{ ml/dL} + 0.186 \text{ ml/dL}$
$C_{\bar{v}}O_2 = .6(10 \times 1.34) + (32 \text{ mmHg} \times 0.0031)$
$8.14 \text{ ml/dL} = 8.04 \text{ ml/dL} + 0.099 \text{ ml/dL}$

With the above information, the $\frac{\dot{Q}_{sp}}{\dot{Q}_T}$ can now be calculated:

$$\frac{\dot{Q}_{sp}}{\dot{Q}_T} = \frac{14.57\ ^{ml}/_{dL} - 12.52\ ^{ml}/_{dL}}{14.57\ ^{ml}/_{dL} - 8.14\ ^{ml}/_{dL}}$$

$$= \frac{2.05\ ^{ml}/_{dL}}{6.43\ ^{ml}/_{dL}}$$

$$= 0.1388 \times 100$$

$$\frac{\dot{Q}_{sp}}{\dot{Q}_T} = 32\%$$

87. a
88. e
89. d
90. d
91. c
92. a, d
93. b, d
94. b
95. a
96. a
97. d
98. e
99. e
100. b
101. c
102. a, c, d, e, g, h, j, k
103. e
104. a, e
105. e
106. $DO_2 = 1000$

$C_aO_2 = 18$

$$\dot{Q}_T = \frac{DO_2}{C_aO_2\,(10)} = \frac{1000}{180}$$

$$\dot{Q}_T = 5.5\ ^{L}/_{min}$$

107. b
108. a
109. d
110. c
111. a
112. b
113. d
114. e
115. c
116. b
117. a. ↓
    b. ↑
    c. <—>
    d. <—>
118. a
119. b
120. a
121. a
122. c
123. a
124. a
125. e
126. c
127. d
128. c
129. d
130. a
131. e
132. a, c
133. a
134. a
135. b
136. d
137. c
138. a
139. b
140. e